The Best Guide to Allergy

THE
BEST
GUIDE TO
ALLERGY

NATHAN D. SCHULTZ, MD
ALLAN V. GIANNINI, MD
TERRANCE T. CHANG, MD
AND DIANE C. WONG

THIRD EDITION

 HUMANA PRESS • TOTOWA, NEW JERSEY

Dedication

We dedicate this book to our teachers

WILLIAM C. DEAMER, MD
OSCAR L. FRICK, MD

NOTICE: The authors and publisher of this book have, as far as it is possible to do so, taken care to make certain that recommendations regarding treatment and use of drugs are correct and compatible with the standards generally accepted at the time of publication. However, knowledge in allergy is constantly changing. As new information becomes available, changes in treatment and in the use of drugs may become necessary. The reader is urged to consult his or her physician for professional advice in dealing with any serious or potentially serious allergic problem.

Illustrated by Diana Reiss

© 1994 by Humana Press Inc.
999 Riverview Drive, Suite 208
Totowa, NJ 07512

Printed in the United States of America   10 9 8 7 6 5 4 3 2

Library of Congress Cataloging-in-Publication Data
The Best guide to allergy / Nathan D. Schultz . . . [et al.]. -- 3rd ed.
    p.   cm.
    Includes index.
    ISBN 0-89603-283-3
    1. Previous ed. published: New York : Appleton-Century-Crofts,
1981. 2. Allergy--Popular works. I. Schultz, Nathan D.
RC584.B45 1994
616.97--dc20   94-11376
                                                            CIP

Preface

This is a new and completely updated edition of *The Best Guide to Allergy*. We hope and believe that in its pages we have successfully provided clear directions through the often dense forest of information about allergies and asthma. New data generated by the powerful techniques of modern biomedical research springs up rapidly, and much has changed since the previous edition. *The Best Guide to Allergy* will help you through this wealth of information, providing perspectives that will allow you, the allergy sufferer, to safely navigate the complex maze of freeways and byways that characterize most allergic disease manifestations.

Everyone suffering from allergies and asthma very much needs to be well-informed in order to make correct and rational decisions about the optimal care of his or her health. The answers you will find here are our very best responses to those questions about allergy and asthma most frequently asked of us by our patients, our families, and our friends.

The health care information we offer in *The Best Guide to Allergy* largely emerges from the research carried out in university medical schools in the United States and around the world. In every era full and clear knowledge has dispelled mystery and puzzlement—after all, we know that despots hold on to their power by keeping entire populations enslaved in ignorance. We are thus confident you will gain real control over your allergies and their symptoms as you read and understand our book.

In all that we write here, we have carefully endeavored to avoid the traps of fads and of overly simplified cure-all explanations, benefiting from the examples afforded by some of the eminent physicians who taught us years ago at the University of California at San Francisco. Thus, we are particularly grateful for our training in the scientific method to the world renowned and brilliant Dr. Oscar L. Frick, and in the artfully quizzical approach of Dr. William C. Deamer, who was suspicious of those healers who marched on "unhampered" by knowledge. Though the language we employ is largely nontechnical, the medical concepts we advance are well-founded in established scientific principles.

In addition to our strong adherence to the principles of scientific medicine, we have not hesitated to include information on new self-help approaches and to revive appropriate ideas and methods from certain ancient healing arts, including such mindfulness exercises as meditation, yoga, and tai-chi, where these have been shown to be helpful to patients.

The word "doctor" has common linguistic origins with "teacher"; with mindful vision and participation, we believe that you, the patient, can also become a teacher. We, the physicians, know that we are always learning much more from you than you imagine. Clearly, we must continue to listen carefully—and you must insist on this. But beyond that, we strongly recommend that you become an activist in behalf of your own health and its best care. Make demands. Don't be satisfied and quieted by statements without explanations. Trust your own inner intuitions. In short, we have striven, in *The Best Guide to Allergy*, to help you avoid becoming a victim of your allergy and asthma, or even of the medical system from which you seek help.

To sum up: *The Best Guide to Allergy* offers a practical, everyday approach to alleviating your allergy and asthma. We feel we have put together a body of hard scientific knowledge that, together with your intuitive understanding, can truly constitute a caring guide to the usually basic, but sometimes difficult, regimens that are necessary to sustain you in good health. We hope to help you and those you care for conquer your allergies completely, and so lead a fuller and more enjoyable life.

ACKNOWLEDGMENTS: Special thanks to our patients, to our publisher, Tom Lanigan, and to Betsy Savery, RN, whose expertise was invaluable in the preparation of this new edition. Betsy worked with the individual personalities and writing styles of the several authors, who truly appreciate her bright and energetic assistance.

Through the long and often intense periods of preparation needed to create this work, we experienced a mutual exchange of love and closeness among our four different families. This was a special gift for which we are all deeply grateful.

Contents

1

What Is Allergy?

WHAT IS ALLERGY?

Allergy is the abnormal response of your immune system to substances that do not elicit such adverse reactions in normal individuals. The symptoms of the hyperreactive immune response that commonly mark an allergy may include any of the following, either singly or in combination: sneezing, running nose, and congestion; watery and itchy eyes; wheezing; redness and itching of the affected area; and many other troublesome irritations.

If you are allergic to a substance, you are likely to experience some of the adverse reactions mentioned above when exposed to even small amounts of the allergen—amounts so apparently minor that, for example, there have been reports of fatalities from the odor of fish. Most reported life-threatening reactions come from peanuts, which are found in trace amounts in prepared foods and often unknowingly ingested. We ourselves have recently been asked to investigate the case of a ten-year-old boy in northern California who died after eating a single bite of cake with peanut butter icing. In a similar case, two New England college students died, not long ago, after eating a restaurant's "house special" chili made with a "secret ingredient"—peanut butter. The allergic person is often dramatically affected by minute quantities of a substance, whereas even large amounts of the same allergen cause no adverse reaction in nonallergic people. Penicillin is a good example. Well-known as a substance that usually heals by killing bacteria, it also sometimes kills those with unsuspected allergies to it.

DO I HAVE AN ALLERGY OR AN INTOLERANCE?

Intolerance is an unpleasant reaction to a substance that does not involve the immune system, although it often produces some of the symptoms of an allergy. Depending on the particular substance, intolerance may be either almost universal or relatively rare. Most antihistamines, for example, can cause you some drowsiness, but if antihistamines make you excessively sleepy, you are intolerant of them, not allergic to them. If you and your physician are trying to identify your allergens, be sure to keep a careful record of any serious adverse reactions you experience whether they seem to be caused by allergy or not. With regard to foods, for example, milk lactose *intolerance* (which produces exaggerated quantities of gas or diarrhea) can be very uncomfortable, whereas milk *allergy* in the extreme can be fatal (by causing anaphylaxis). Classic examples of other food intolerances are the relatively common inability to digest beans that results in bloating and gas, and the relatively uncommon intestinal damage (diarrhea and ulceration) caused by gluten (found in wheat and other grains) in susceptible individuals.

Even the symptoms of asthma can be a manifestation of intolerance, with no immune allergic mechanism. A significant number of asthmatic patients are intolerant of the sulfite preservatives generally used in such foods as dried fruits, powdered potatoes, wine, and sometimes in salad bars. Ingestion of these foods causes severe asthmatic reactions because sulfur dioxide fumes are produced in the stomach, rise into the airway, and trigger asthma. One unfortunate sulfite-sensitive asthmatic died after exposure to sulfur dioxide fumes while touring a volcano in Hawaii. More recently, the Environmental Protection Agency (EPA) has determined that particulate air pollution—plain old soot—is particularly dangerous to asthmatics and can precipitate life-threatening attacks.

Understanding whether any given reaction to a substance that you experience is caused by either allergy or intolerance will help your physician choose an effective or safe drug for your future treatment. Sometimes it is difficult to determine from the description of a particular reaction to the symptoms of a substance whether it was a true allergy, an intolerance, or perhaps even an unrelated hormonal or nervous system reaction. The history might be that you sometimes develop flushing after eating, though no specific food "stands out" in your food diary. Or you may feel itchy after taking a variety of drugs completely unrelated to each other.

But all is not confusion. There is a blood test that can help document that you have sustained an acute allergic reaction. A chemical called tryptase is released during a true allergic reaction and can be detected for up to 8 hours after the episode. If there is a high level of tryptase in your blood immediately after you suffer a reaction to something, your allergist is on the right track in investigating thoroughly for an allergic cause.

How Common Is Allergy?

The latest statistics from the National Institutes of Health report that there are 43 million Americans with allergies, some 17% of our population. Allergy is thus one of the most common health problems, and everyone knows someone who suffers from allergy. There are 10 million asthmatics in this country, and this number is increasing. The prevalance of asthma increased 29% from 1980 to 1987 (*see* NIH publication nos. 79–387 [1979] and 91–3042 [1991]). Almost 18 million Americans suffer from hay fever alone, and another 14 million are afflicted with other allergic diseases. In short, about one out of five people has an allergy.

Other countries report somewhat different statistics on various allergies, which may reflect racial (genetic) or environmental differences—or possibly just different reporting or treatment practices.

How Can I Tell Whether I Have An Allergy?

Classically, allergy is manifested by your immediate, acute reaction to a substance that is inhaled, eaten, touched, or injected. It may also be expressed by more gradually appearing symptoms in your nose, eyes, or chest, such as congestion, itchiness, or wheezing.

A word of caution! Such symptoms are not always allergic in origin and other causes should also be considered. Serious infections—such as herpes of the eyes, parts of toys or food particles lodged in the nose or chest, and infectious bronchitis—all produce symptoms that can masquerade as allergies. There is considerable overlap, and your allergist can help you sort out your symptoms by taking a history, a physical exam, and testing.

What Are Allergens?

Allergens are the actual substances (usually proteins) that elicit your allergic immune response (*see* box on next page for some of the well-recognized allergens).

SOME WELL-RECOGNIZED ALLERGENS

- **Foods:** peanuts, nuts, fish, eggs, milk, chocolate
- **Inhalant allergens:** house dust mites; mold spores; cat and dog dander and saliva; birds and feathers; cockroaches; pollen from trees, weeds and grasses
- **Contact allergens:** poison oak, poison ivy, and nickel (found in jewelry), latex rubber, and cosmetic ingredients, all of which can cause allergic reactions that occur mainly in the skin
- **Drugs:** penicillin, sulfa, aspirin, and ibuprofen
- **Insect venoms:** honeybee, wasp, yellow jacket, hornet, and fire ant
- **Chemicals:** MDI and TDI-diisocyanates (plastics and paints)

WHAT IS ANAPHYLAXIS?

Anaphylaxis refers to any type of immediate—and sometimes severely life-threatening—allergic reaction. The reaction may be limited to a few hives or it may be generalized, with wheezing and shock (loss of blood pressure). The stings of insects can result in anaphylaxis. Many substances, but especially drugs and foods, may cause an acute anaphylactic reaction. Penicillin is the most common drug offender and is much more likely to cause anaphylaxis when injected than when taken orally. Our most careful patients have unwittingly encountered severe difficulty by eating cookies containing nuts or peanuts that were not so labeled.

Anaphylaxis can be associated with both menstrual cycles and exercise. Women are known to be more susceptible to these reactions toward the end of their normal menstrual cycles, when progesterone levels in the blood are increased. For some still undiscovered reason, a mild allergy to such foods as celery or shrimp may become fatal when the victim exercises shortly after eating the food.

Many deaths have resulted from untreated severe anaphylaxis. Mild, limited anaphylactic reactions can be treated with antihistamines (for example, Benadryl, Chlor-Trimeton), but

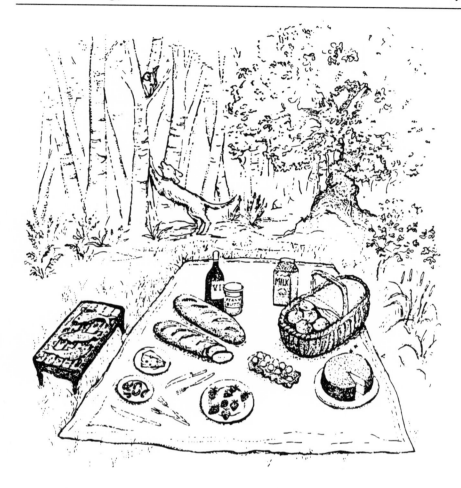

The allergy picnic. Twenty potential allergens: cheese, milk, chocolate, eggs, tomatoes, bees, wine, wheat, peanut butter, fish, shrimp, poison oak, dog and cat dander, oak and birch trees, timothy grass, plantain grass, and bluegrass.

severe, generalized reactions require adrenalin by injection. Oxygen therapy may also be necessary when breathing is obstructed. The administration of prednisone or other steroids may prevent recurrence when the offending agent is expected to remain in the body for hours or days.

If you suffer anaphylaxis or other serious symptoms of allergy, you should arrange an allergy consultation promptly in order to identify the responsible agent. Persons diagnosed as being at risk for recurrent, severe anaphylactic reactions should always carry lifesaving injectable adrenalin. Ask your physician to prescribe an EpiPen or Ana-Kit and instruct you and your family in its use. Most deaths from food anaphylaxis occur when emergency adrenalin has not been used.

WHAT EXACTLY IS HAPPENING IN AN ALLERGIC REACTION?

The basic mechanism of an allergic reaction involves four elements: the antibody, the mast cells, the mediators (chemical messengers) such as histamine, and the body organs that are affected. When an allergen enters your body through the mucous membranes of the respiratory or digestive systems, or by injection, it is carried to lymph tissue, including the tonsils and lymph nodes, where it comes into contact with lymphocytes (a type of white blood cell), which then produce the primary antibody of allergy, immunoglobulin E (IgE). Recent evidence indicates that a subclass of another antibody (IgG) may also play a minor role in the allergic response. The IgE produced by your lymphocytes then attaches to your mast cells, which are present in various organs, especially the nose, lungs, gastrointestinal tract, and skin. With subsequent exposures to the allergen, your now-sensitized mast cells become excited and release such mediators as histamines, leukotrienes, and platelet-activating factor that then circulate through the body and trigger your allergic symptoms. A very recently discovered mediator of allergic reactions is nitric oxide, which should not be confused with nitrous oxide, a form of anesthesia commonly known as laughing gas. In response to the allergic reaction, nitric oxide gas is rapidly released from the lining of the blood vessels causing them to dilate, and leading to a pooling of blood in the abdomen, loss of blood pressure, and consequent shock.

Special white blood cells, called eosinophils, and polymorphonuclear leukocytes also play important roles in amplifying the allergic reaction by helping produce the inflammation attending most allergic responses. This recently developed concept that the result of the allergic reaction is inflammation has led to new understandings and treatments in asthma. Anti-inflammatory agents such as inhaled steroids (Aerobid), cromolyn (Intal), or nedocromil (Tilade) are now seen as essential, along with such bronchodilators as albuterol, for effective treatment of asthma.

Certain chemicals released by the nerve endings of the bronchial tubes are also known to trigger asthmatic spasms and nasal discharge; these include the neurotransmitter substance P. Thus, when you eat hot peppers, you experience the sensation of burning and your nose clogs immediately. Capsaicin—the "hot" chemical found in hot peppers—causes the mucous membranes to release substance P on contact, and this then produces the inflammation you experience.

WHAT IS CLINICAL IMMUNOLOGY?

The field of clinical immunology is closely allied with that of allergy since both study and treat the immune system and the phenomenon of immunity. Clinical immunology is the scientific backbone of allergy medicine.

Immunity is basically the ability your body has to protect itself from foreign substances. If we had no immunity, other living cells and viruses would invade our bodies; germs, fungi, and parasites would soon destroy our tissues. And not completely surprisingly, the newest explanation for the induction of labor and delivery is that the fetus ultimately loses its protection from immune rejection, becomes seen by the mother's immune system as a mass of invading foreign cells, and must then be rejected. This special ability of the human body to recognize its own cells while rejecting and killing foreign cells is truly an amazing biological phenomenon.

Immune protection comes from our white blood cells, called the *lymphocytes*. There are two types, T lymphocytes and B lymphocytes. The T lymphocytes are subdivided into various kinds. Some T cells surround and kill invading bacteria, viruses, fungi, or transplanted cells by releasing toxic substances that destroy

---

GAMMA GLOBULINS

- **IgG**, the most common antibody class
    Responsible for long-lasting protection after vaccinations
    Protects against tetanus, hepatitis, diphtheria, and so on
- **IgM**
    Rapid but short-lasting protection from infection
    The earliest protective response
    An early indicator of hepatitis infection
- **IgA**
    Present in blood, in nasal and gastric secretions, and in
        breast milk
    Provide the first line of antibody defense at mucous mem-
        branes
    One in 200 allergy patients lack IgA, which renders them
        more prone to respiratory infections
- **IgE**, the primary class of allergy antibodies
    Provide protection against parasites
    Abnormal overproduction is the primary factor leading to
        allergic response

---

their biological machinery. Some T cells secrete chemical factors
that recruit other types of white blood cells to help neutralize or
destroy substances foreign to your body. And special helper T
cells (CD4⁺ cells) stimulate the immune system itself to increase
its defense.

B lymphocytes secrete soluble proteins called *antibodies*.
Antibodies have the ability to recognize the presence of foreign
proteins that belong to either infecting organisms or allergenic
substances. The active part of the antibody is a three-dimensional mirror image of the specific foreign protein. First, the
antibody finds the foreign protein on the germ or virus, or in the
allergens, and then simply attaches to it. Once combined with
their specific antibodies, these foreign materials are targeted
either for easy ingestion by your white blood cells or for destruction by the blood substance called *complement*.

Antibodies are found in your blood serum and are divided
into several classes commonly known as *gamma globulins* (*see* box).

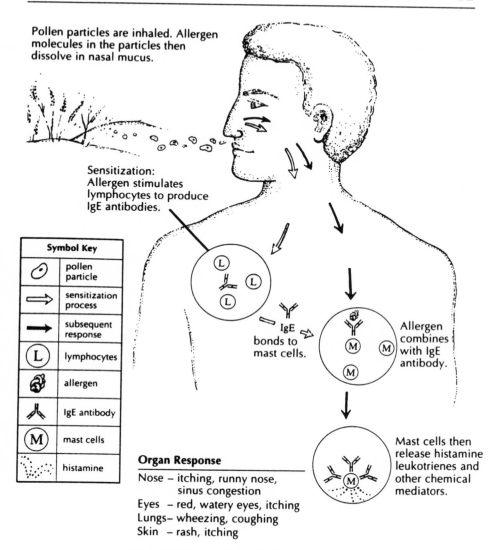

Pollen particles are inhaled. Allergen molecules in the particles then dissolve in nasal mucus.

Sensitization: Allergen stimulates lymphocytes to produce IgE antibodies.

Symbol Key	
⊘	pollen particle
⇒	sensitization process
→	subsequent response
Ⓛ	lymphocytes
🦠	allergen
⅄	IgE antibody
Ⓜ	mast cells
⋯	histamine

IgE bonds to mast cells.

Allergen combines with IgE antibody.

Mast cells then release histamine leukotrienes and other chemical mediators.

Organ Response

Nose – itching, runny nose, sinus congestion
Eyes – red, watery eyes, itching
Lungs – wheezing, coughing
Skin – rash, itching

Sensitization and the allergic response.

People whose bodies do not produce an adequate supply of antibodies suffer from recurrent severe infections, and those whose T lymphocytes are deficient or reduced in number are especially susceptible to viral, fungal, and parasitic infections, as well as cancer. T lymphocytes can kill tumor cells in addition to the cells of transplanted organs. Clinical immunologists, therefore, are active in AIDS and cancer treatment and research, and in transplant surgery, as well as in allergy itself.

CAN MY ALLERGIES CHANGE OVER THE YEARS?

Yes, they can. Symptoms may become worse or better; sensitivities to new allergens may develop while reactions to previous ones disappear. For example, an infant may exhibit allergic symptoms of eczema from cow's milk and eggs. These food problems can vanish for some within a few years, but they might also be replaced by nasal congestion and sneezing from house dust, molds, or cat dander. Wheezing, along with nasal symptoms, may develop within a short time. If symptoms now become worse during the spring, a developing pollen allergy is suspected.

In childhood, spontaneous remission is more common with asthma than with nasal symptoms. Food allergies are usually more of a problem during the early years of life, resolving or becoming far less serious as time goes on.

Avoidance of your specific allergens over many years may therefore result in the reduction of those sensitivities. But the best control of your allergy can be achieved only with an allergy care program that includes skin testing and immunotherapy.

CAN ALLERGY BE PREVENTED?

The tendency to develop allergies is inherited, but medical intervention may control the actual clinical appearance of symptoms. Vigorous research into the prevention of allergic disease is currently being carried out by pediatric allergists in many medical schools. All the answers are not yet in, but several guidelines have already been established. Allergic parents-to-be, for example, would be wise to choose breast feeding for their newborn. Among other benefits, this avoids the infant's ingestion of large amounts of the frequently allergenic proteins in cow's milk. A word of caution. Food allergens can also be present in breast milk. Nursing mothers from allergic families should clearly avoid eating excessive amounts of such allergenic foods as nuts, chocolate, and eggs (and perhaps even avoid cow's milk).

The development of specific allergies is related to repeated exposure to the allergens. The presence of animals in the house increases the likelihood of early sensitization. If allergic parents keep cats or dogs in their homes, they are asking for trouble.

How Do Skin Tests Work?

Skin testing is currently the best practical method for detecting the allergens to which you may be sensitive. There are two methods: scratching or pricking the skin, and intradermal injection. Allergists initially perform scratch tests, a technique that usually reveals the majority of significant allergies. Skin tests by intradermal injections are necessary only when suspected sensitivities to inhalants, venoms, and drugs are not revealed by the scratch or prick tests.

The purpose of all these tests is to determine—by introducing a small amount of the suspected allergen into the skin—whether you have an allergy to a *specific* substance. Within a few minutes, the presence or absence of a local reaction that produces redness or swelling becomes apparent. Any significant such reaction indicates the presence of the allergy antibody (IgE), and thus a possible allergy to the tested allergen.

Which Skin Tests Are the Most Reliable?

Skin tests for specific pollens, animal danders, house dust mites, and molds are the most reliable and useful types. Recently, excellent venom extracts for bee sting allergy skin testing have become available. Skin tests for foods are sometimes helpful. Finally, testing for inhaled "chemical allergies" has not yet been demonstrated to be a valid diagnostic tool.

Will Skin Tests Tell Me How Severe My Allergies Are?

Only when properly interpreted can allergy skin tests predict the severity of your allergic reactions. If you experience severe symptoms during the ragweed season, you are more likely to have strongly positive skin test reactions to the ragweed test extract, with high degrees of swelling and redness. Since skin

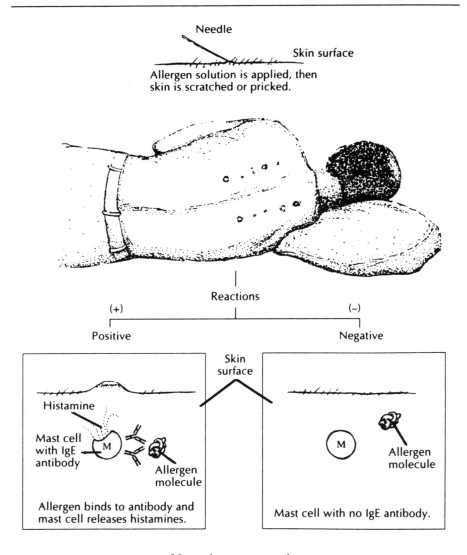

How skin tests work.

tests reflect the amount of IgE present in your skin, their results also generally correlate with the allergic responses of your lungs and eyes. Nevertheless, some people with only moderate reactions and low levels of allergy antibodies may experience severe symptoms because their mucous membranes are exquisitely sensitive to even the smallest amounts of allergy antibody. And just occasionally, skin tests are positive when no underlying allergy or allergy symptoms are present.

Your allergist must carefully correlate your history and skin test results. Treatment with allergy injections should never be based on skin tests alone.

CAN I HAVE ALLERGIES WHEN ALL MY TESTS ARE NEGATIVE?

Yes. Nevertheless, allergy skin testing is very reliable for the diagnosis of allergy to pollens of grasses, trees, and weeds, house dust mites, certain molds, and animals such as cats, dogs, and birds. Allergists currently use a new generation of standardized skin test materials (as well as treatment extracts), assuring high quality; nevertheless, some tests are not as reliable as others. The quality of dog extract test material can vary and the scratch/prick skin test will sometimes be negative in a patient who is actually allergic to dogs. A subsequent intradermal test is often necessary when this type of false-negative result is suspected.

Food skin testing is often misleading. If a food allergy causes an immediate reaction with the ingestion of only small amounts of the suspect food, the skin test is usually positive. If a person is sensitive only to a large amount of the food in question when taken over a prolonged period, the skin test may be negative. The explanation for a negative skin test in the face of allergy is that the skin-tested material contains only the undigested or native food allergen. In fact, current research points to the digested breakdown products of suspect foods as the actual allergens. It seems likely that better test substances for many foods will become available in the near future.

Antihistamines, especially hydroxyzine (Atarax) and astemizole (Hismanal), may depress reactions to skin tests for prolonged periods of time and may result in false-negative test results. Thus you should discontinue most antihistamines at least five to seven days prior to your skin tests. Hismanal may depress skin tests for two months after the last dose and will cause your tests to miss significant allergens. Some antidepressant medications, as well as certain medications used for ulcers, may suppress skin tests. Be sure to check with your allergist. It is not necessary to avoid decongestants. Steroids (cortisone, prednisone), theophylline preparations, and adrenalin-like medicines (Alupent, Proventil-Ventolin, Brethine) do not affect skin testing and may be used up to the time of this procedure.

ARE THERE OTHER TESTS FOR ALLERGY?

Yes, there are. Your allergy specialist can usually tell you about most of your allergy problems without special laboratory tests, but if the problem is complex or puzzling, lab tests may be helpful. Two of these tests are:

1. Microscopic examination for "allergy cells" (*eosinophils*) in your nasal mucus, bronchial secretions, and blood. Quantities of these cells are commonly elevated in nasal allergies and allergic asthma.
2. RAST (radioallergosorbent test) measures the amount of allergen-specific IgE in your blood. Although this test detects specific antibodies, it is not as sensitive as skin testing. With RAST testing alone, some of your allergies may be missed. Moreover, the use of the RAST test has several other limitations, including the number of test allergens available and its high cost. RAST is helpful to confirm and document your severe food allergies when skin testing might be dangerous. Be sure that IgE RAST testing is ordered. IgG RAST tests should usually be considered experimental and will not at this point help you sort out your food allergies. If RAST tests are used, be sure that they are done by a qualified laboratory. In rare cases of generalized skin rashes, such as severe eczema or psoriasis, RAST tests are particularly important and helpful because an adequate skin surface for scratch tests is not available.

WHICH DISORDERS ARE CAUSED BY ALLERGIES?

Hay fever, asthma, hives, and eczema are the clinical disorders most often caused by allergies. At times, stomachaches, headaches (migraine), leg and joint pains, excessive fatigue and

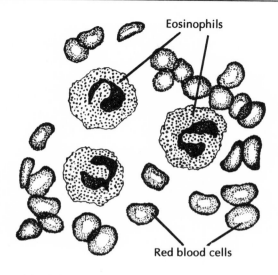

Eosinophils—"allergy cells"—in the blood.

irritability, pallor, and dark circles under the eyes are attributable to allergy. Cases of enuresis (bed wetting) have also been reported as associated with allergy.

Do Allergic People Catch More Colds?

Yes, patients with allergy manifest more frequent swelling of their nasal passages and sinus cavities than nonallergics. When such swellings block the normal drainage of secretions, bacterial infections develop much more easily in the blocked paranasal sinus cavities and in the middle ear.

I've Had My Dogs All My Life. How Can I Be Allergic to Them?

The tendency to develop a particular allergy (for example, to dogs) is inherited at birth. Often, a particular activating event—such as a viral infection or exposure to an excess of an allergen—will "turn on" your largely dormant allergy, after which that response will continue strongly. Frequently the triggering event is not at all apparent to the allergy sufferer. And when incidentally exposed to dogs, you may well not manifest any of the typical allergy symptoms, such as sneezing or wheezing, for many years. Moreover, you may not have recognized the appearance of such subtle symptoms as nasal congestion or a slight cough when occasionally exposed to them. These minimal symptoms are commonly ignored or taken for granted for many years before being recognized as having been caused by an allergic reaction.

DOES TOBACCO SMOKE WORSEN AN ALLERGY?

Tobacco smoke is an irritant as well as a carcinogen, and not an allergen. But tobacco workers may develop an allergy to the tobacco leaf itself. Here, the lung's reaction to smoke produces irreversible damage, whereas the lung's reaction to allergens such as cat fur is reversible, however miserable your symptoms may make you.

Many nonsmokers feel harrassed (if not overtly sickened) by exposure to second-hand smoke, which is now known to cause respiratory symptoms similar to those of allergy. Often you cough and wheeze, your nose is congested, and your eyes burn. If you suffer from allergies to begin with, this second-hand smoke is even more dangerous. Irritant exposure can flare both asthma and nasal allergies, as well as actually increasing the frequency of bronchial infections. This is especially true in children. *Parents should know that, if they smoke, their very young children also smoke.*

HOW DO VIRUSES AND SMOKING CAUSE ALLERGY?

Viral infections and exposure to tobacco smoke can actually cause an increase in your production of the special IgE allergy antibodies, which are then directed against such specific allergens as house dust mites, cats, and grass pollen. Recent research has shown that this mechanism is in fact responsible for allergy sensitization in infants—resulting in their development of both asthma and hay fever. Similar research has demonstrated that, in some children, a severe gastrointestinal infection allows food allergens to enter the body more readily through the gut wall, enter the lymph system, and thus induce the allergic response.

SOURCES OF HIV TRANSMISSION

- Intimate sexual contact with exchange of semen or vaginal secretions
- Intravenous drug use
- Nontested blood transfusions
- Accidental contaminated-needle punctures
- Infants born to HIV-infected mothers

If you are going to have a baby, we strongly recommend that you no longer allow anyone to smoke in your house. During your pregnancy, your cat (or dog, bird, etc.) should be removed from the house months before the new baby arrives, and the entire house should be thoroughly cleaned and vacuumed so your infant is not brought home to face a large residual amount of cat allergen. If one or both parents is allergic, especially to cats, the development of a cat allergy by your new baby upon exposure is very likely unless these measures are taken.

You can also protect your infant by avoiding exposure to tobacco smoke and by avoiding crowded environments where your infant will be exposed to airborne viruses.

WHAT SHOULD I KNOW ABOUT AIDS?

AIDS is caused by a virus called HIV (human immunodeficiency virus) that infects patients through body fluids—blood products, semen, and vaginal secretions (*see* box).

No family is immune to AIDS. The latest statistics from the Centers for Disease Control, United States Department of Health and Human Services in Atlanta, show that in many communities in this country HIV disease is the leading cause of death among men and women in the 25–44-year age group. In this young population, HIV accounts for 14% of deaths in men and 4% in women. The prevention of AIDS with changing sexual practices has already been significantly effective in the gay population, but unfortunately, this important message of prevention is not reaching as many young men and women as it should.

How Does AIDS Damage the Immune System?

In AIDS, a special group of your lymphocyte white blood cells first becomes infected with the HIV virus. These helper T cells—known as CD4⁺ cells—are necessary for normal immunity. The HIV virus, which eventually leads to AIDS, reproduces itself inside of your infected T cells, killing these cells, after which the newly generated copies of the virus move on to infect and kill still more CD4⁺ cells. As your CD4⁺ T cell levels fall—especially when the count drops below 500—you become increasingly susceptible to severe and unusual infections, as well as to cancer and neurological changes.

As allergists, we see patients who are infected with HIV. They suffer from increased numbers of sinus infections, increased allergy symptoms in general, and frequent, severe yeast infections in the throat, as well as in the vagina. Allergy to antibiotics, especially to the sulfa drugs used in the treatment of *Pneumocystis pneumonia*, is far more common in AIDS patients and we are often asked to desensitize so that treatment can continue.

Should My Allergist Know I Am HIV Positive?

Yes. If you are HIV positive, let your allergist know so that you can be counseled and otherwise made aware of potential problems. For those uncertain of their HIV status, HIV is diagnosed by a blood test that detects antibodies to the virus. But since there is a delay (weeks to months) between the time of infection and the appearance of the antibodies and a diagnostically positive HIV test, you should be tested periodically, particularly if you are in a high risk group—gay or bisexual men, intravenous drug users, or sexual partners of these persons.

2

Hay Fever

2 Hay Fever

What Is Vasomotor Rhinitis?
Does a Deviated Septum Complicate Allergy?
Is Nasal Endoscopy Helpful?
What About Kids Who Put Things in Their Noses?
Where Do Nasal Polyps Originate?

WHAT IS HAY FEVER?

Hay fever is a common allergy characterized by an array of symptoms involving the nose, eyes, throat, ears, and skin. These symptoms include nasal congestion, sneezing, and production of clear, watery discharge; conjunctival irritation with runny, itchy eyes; throat soreness and irritation from postnasal drip; ear pain and the feeling of ear pressure; and generalized fatigue, irritability, and headaches. Hay fever sufferers may also have concurrent asthma with its wheezing and coughing. Hay fever's symptoms can occur during a specific season, such as spring, continuously throughout the year, or even sporadically without any pattern.

Hay fever is an old English term originally describing symptoms experienced during hay pitching time. These symptoms were often so severe that the afflicted person actually felt feverish; hence, the term "hay fever." Now we know that the symptoms are caused by almost all airborne pollens and mold spores, as well as by hay or cut grass itself. Hay fever is more properly called allergic rhinoconjunctivitis.

Hay fever occurs in individuals who have been previously sensitized by an allergen such as grass pollen. With subsequent exposures to the allergen, the body's immune system activates the IgE machinery. This interaction between specific IgE allergic antibodies and the allergen(s) leads to the emergence of hay fever symptoms.

IS HAY FEVER SEASONAL?

Not always. Most persons use the term to refer to clearly defined seasonal difficulties. These generally include nasal congestion, excessive clear nasal secretions, sneezing, itchiness of the nose, watery and itchy eyes, and sometimes itchiness of the ears and throat.

The pollen season varies in different parts of the United States. Ragweed is a severe problem in the East, Midwest, and South during the late summer. Grass is the strongest allergen in the West, and pollinates primarily during the months of April, May, and June. Other important allergens, which may vary in different regions, include the pollens of juniper, cedar, cypress,

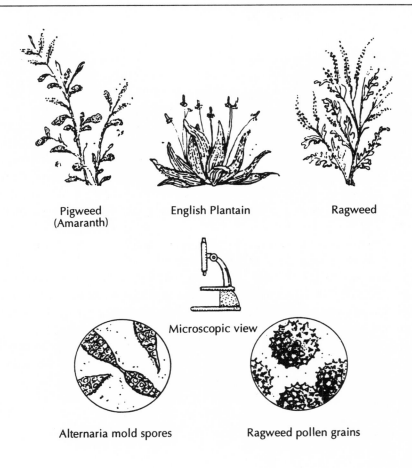

Pigweed   English Plantain   Ragweed
(Amaranth)

Microscopic view

Alternaria mold spores   Ragweed pollen grains

Weeds, molds, and pollens.

and the mold spores of Alternaria, Cladosporium (Hormodendrum), and Aspergillus.

WHAT IS THE POLLEN COUNT TODAY?

For today, no one knows for sure since pollen and mold spore counts represent the average counts for the *previous* 24 hours. The counts are reported as the number of pollen grains or spores per cubic meter of air over a 24-hour period. The samples are

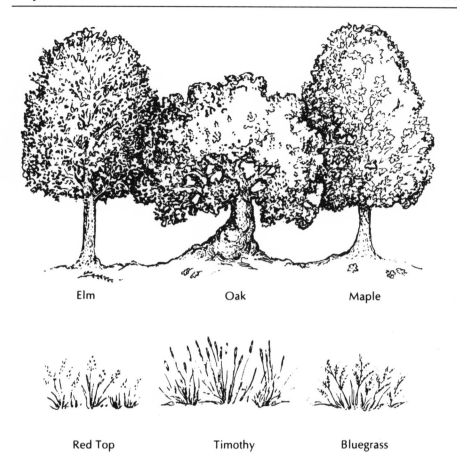

| Elm | Oak | Maple |

| Red Top | Timothy | Bluegrass |

Trees and grasses.

usually collected on a small microscope slide or spinning rod; they are then stained and visually identified under the microscope. Placement of the pollen collecting device is very important because surrounding buildings, wind currents, nearby forests, and even its height from the ground can dramatically affect the pollen and spore count. So, when you hear the pollen count on the radio or see it in the newspaper, you cannot predict what will happen *today*—there are too many variables. Thus if it is raining today, obviously the pollen counts will be down.

POLLEN GRAINS OR MOLD SPORES PER CUBIC METER OF AIR OVER 24 HOURS				
	Low	Moderate	High	Very High
Grass	0–5	5–20	20–200	>200
Trees	0–15	15–90	90–1500	>1500
Weeds	0–10	10–50	50–500	>500
Molds	0–900	900–2500	2500–25,000	>25,000

The usefulness of pollen counts comes over a long period. You can "see how the season is going" and have an explanation for your symptoms. Pollen counts also help the allergist know that the skin test correlates with clinical history, a fact critical in deciding whether allergy shots are needed. You may see pollen counts reported in the various media as low, moderate, or high. This designation is usually a reflection of the range of counts seen for that pollen in your particular area. For the sake of comparison, according to the American Academy of Allergy and Immunology Pollen and Mold Network, these designations may be interpreted with the parameters as shown in the above box.

How Can Pollen and Mold Spore Counts Help Me?

Recent research has shown that beginning your antihistamine and other allergy medications before your symptoms start up and then taking them regularly during the season provides the most relief. This year's pollen counts help make the present season predictable. Looking at last year's pollen count data will suggest when to begin taking your prescribed preventive nasal and asthma sprays; ideally, a few weeks before the season starts. Once they've flared and become primed for your allergies, your symptoms are much more difficult to control.

What Is Rose Fever?

"Rose fever" is the folk term for spring hay fever. The term originated from the observation that people became congested and sneezed when roses came into bloom. Actually, the pollen of ornate flowers rarely causes hay fever because it is sticky and does not easily get into the air. Birds and such insects as bees are attracted to the flowers and carry the sticky pollen away on their bodies to fertilize other flowering plants; thus, the meaning of the phrase, "the birds and the bees." If you smell flowers up close, of course, problems can result. So, remember, hay fever or allergy-inducing plants rarely have conspicuous, large, beautiful, or fragrant flowers.

DOES GEOGRAPHY AFFECT ALLERGY DRAMATICALLY?

Ragweed is a major hay fever plant east of the Rockies, while the western varieties of this weed produce relatively little pollen. At altitudes above 5000 feet there are *relatively* few allergenic pollens. Areas with cold, freezing winters have very short hay fever seasons. Near the arctic circle in Alaska and Norway, birch pollen produces a short, but heavy hay fever season. For decades Easterners moved to the southwest to avoid ragweed hay fever; but now allergenic grasses and trees introduced by those migrating to the area thrive with the warmth and increasing irrigation. Bermuda grass and mulberry trees have brought hay fever even to Tucson, Arizona.

Pacific islanders from Hawaii and the Philippines have more problems with allergy in California than at home. There are fewer wind pollinated plants in the tropical islands. The lush flowers of Kauai do not cause hay fever. In general, wind-borne pollens blow out to the sea and insect pollinated plants thrive. Mold, dust mite and dander allergies persist in tropical climates. As a bonus, eczema clears up in the humid tropical climate. *See* box on next page for some tips for travelers.

CAN I HAVE HAY FEVER SYMPTOMS ALL YEAR?

Yes. Your symptoms may persist even throughout the winter months when pollens are no longer present. House dust is the major cause of perennial (year-round) allergic rhinitis. A tiny organism that is best seen with a microscope is the most important allergenic component of house dust—the house dust mite. The concentration and species of the house dust mites varies

---

SOME TIPS FOR TRAVELERS

- Take a supply of your allergy medications with you. Expect the worst and be prepared.
- Seasons vary. Grass pollinates in California in May, in New York in June, and in Sweden in July.
- There is no ragweed in Europe.
- Mite and mold allergy in England—the worst.
- In Ireland, grass makes the Emerald Isle.
- Mediterranean climate and allergy follow each other. California is similar to southern France, Italy, and Israel.
- Birch allergy predominates in the Scandinavian spring.
- Airborne particles of codfish cause respiratory allergies in Norway.
- House dust mites, but not significant pollens, are found in developed Hong Kong.
- Mexico: The coast is clear, but grass and trees predominate inland.

---

with changes in climate in different cities; nevertheless, the genus, Dermatophagoides ("skin eater") is identical throughout the world. It lives on surfaces of mattresses and in carpets, but not on people. Of greater interest, however, is the fact that it feeds on the tiny flecks of human skin that your body constantly sheds, as well as on molds in damp climates. Additionally, cockroaches can be a major cause of allergy symptoms, especially in urban areas. These may be allergy associated, and persistent loss of smell may indicate nasal polyps or chronic sinus infections.

Animal dander and saliva from your cat and dog may also be responsible for your nonseasonal allergies. They are usually the most important causes of allergy in homes with pets.

Finally, mold allergy must be kept in mind—especially in older homes with damp rooms. Mold or mildew may also be found in showers, decks, porches, basements, and house plants. Recent studies also point to straw carpets, woven baskets, vegetable bins, and car and home air conditioners.

Is Mildew Bad for My Allergy and Asthma?

The mold spores released from mildew cause allergy. The exact levels of mold spores needed to cause allergy symptoms are not known; however, you can measure the level of mold spores in different rooms of your home as well as those on your porch. This can be helpful in deciding on the use of specific mold control measures. In allergy research, the concept of colony-forming units is used. Samples from the home are collected on a culture medium and the resulting mold colonies are counted. There are hundreds of species of molds, but relatively few are allergenic. Mold spore counts are generally higher outdoors than indoors. This is particularly true in agricultural areas. Indoor moisture found in bathrooms and basements results in a higher than average spore count for those rooms. The most common indoor allergenic molds are Penicillium and Aspergillus, whereas the most common outdoor molds are Alternaria and Cladosporium. These are found in all areas of the United States. By the way, allergy to Penicillium mold spores has nothing to do with allergy to the antibiotic penicillin. Penicillin is a substance produced by the body of the mold and none of the penicillin itself is found in the airborne spores. A person who reacts on skin testing and clinically to Penicillium spores is not necessarily allergic to the antibiotic.

Have I Lost My Sense of Smell?

You may be unable to smell (or taste your food) when allergies cause severe swelling of the mucosal lining of your nose. The olfactory nerve endings for your sense of smell become blocked by the edema and the excessive secretions produced by your allergy so that the tiny molecules that transmit odor from your food cannot make contact with them. Persistent congestion with an accompanying loss of smell may indicate that your condition has gone beyond allergy as such and that you may have developed nasal polyps or a chronic sinus infection. After receiving appropriate treatment for nasal allergies, patients are often surprised—and delighted—that they can again smell.

SHOULD I BE CONCERNED ABOUT CANCER IN MY NOSE?

Nasopharyngeal cancer may occur in anyone, though it is prevalent chiefly in certain Asian populations. Specifically, Chinese populations from Hong Kong and other areas of Southern China are known to be especially susceptible to this cancer of the interior nose and throat area. Some speculate that there is a causal link with the preservatives—especially nitrates—used in salted fish consumed in large quantities by these populations. Symptoms of decreased smell, bleeding, and irritation, as well as nasal obstruction, that mimic allergies may actually be signs of cancer. A Cantonese adult with fluid in the middle ear should be evaluated by an ear, nose, and throat surgeon as well as an allergist.

DO I HAVE A COLD OR AN ALLERGY IN MY NOSE?

You may indeed have a cold. If your symptoms persist for more than several weeks, however, and if there are no other household members with similar complaints, then you probably have a nasal allergy that is masquerading as a cold. A severe sore throat with muscle aches along with your fever suggest a cold or flu. Sometimes an irritable cough can persist for one to three weeks following a bad cold. The nasal mucosa—the lining of your nose—is characteristically pale or pearly gray with allergy. In addition, a characteristic type of white blood cell, the eosinophil, is often present in your clear allergic nasal secretions. With a cold your mucosa is red and angry-looking, and the secretions are often pale yellow to green. Finally, untreated allergies may predispose people to colds. Repeated colds are indeed infections, but they tend to become more frequent because of the underlying allergic state. Once your allergy is under control, so is the seemingly exaggerated frequency of such infections.

WHY ARE MY EYES RED?

Nasal allergies commonly involve the outer membrane of the eye, the conjunctiva, which, like your nose, contains mast cells. (Remember, the mast cells release histamine when allergies occur.) The released histamine causes swelling by allowing leakage of watery fluid into the tissues surrounding your eye. It also causes the blood vessels in your eyes to dilate, producing their reddish appearance. Rubbing your eyes to relieve the itchiness only adds to the redness. Excessive use of decongestant eye drops may result in persistent red eyes.

You should also consider the possibility that an infection of the conjunctiva may be present. In this case the conjunctiva is also inflamed and the symptoms may be similar to those of allergies. Sometimes thick yellow secretions accumulate. Antibiotic eye drops are then necessary. Chronic redness of your conjunctiva may also indicate the presence of other diseases and should be evaluated by your physician or an ophthalmologist. Steroid or cortisone drops should be used only under the careful supervision of your physician.

WHY DO MY CONTACT LENSES BOTHER ME?

During the pollen season, pollen grains may fly into your eyes and land between the eye and the contact lens. Then, when you blink your eye, you drag the pollen grain over the eye's delicate mucosa, causing a reaction similar to an allergy skin test, and thereby producing redness, tearing, and irritation. Wearing sunglasses will reduce the amount of pollen exposure to the eyes.

Keep in mind the other possible causes of contact lens irritation: sensitivity to the lens solution, especially the preservatives thimerosal and ethylene diamine; and the possibility of an eye infection, which requires the immediate care of a physician.

Giant papillary conjunctivitis is also a complication of contact lens wear. The irritation results from an inflammatory reaction under your eyelids caused by contamination of the contact lenses with protein from the eye itself. This occurs primarily with soft contact lenses, but has also been seen with hard lenses. The treatment is to remove your contact lenses for one month while medicating with 4% cromolyn sodium eye drops formulated by your pharmacist. New lenses are then necessary.

CAN HAY FEVER CAUSE NOSEBLEEDS?

Nosebleeds can occur as a result of trauma from either rubbing or blowing your nose too often or too hard. Nosebleeds also occur because, as nasal secretions dry, they may pull away from and tear the fragile walls of your nostril's blood vessels. Beware of the excessive use of decongestant nasal sprays, which can also contribute to the problem. Use of cortisone nasal sprays can occasionally be associated with nosebleeds. Once a nosebleed begins, it can easily be stopped by tilting your head back at a 45 degree angle and applying direct pressure to the bleeding nostrils. To prevent recurrence of chronic mild nosebleeds, keep your nasal mucosa moist with Vaseline or Bactroban antibacterial ointment or salt water sprays. Call your physician if your nosebleeds remain persistent or profuse.

WHAT ABOUT NASAL SPRAYS?

When nasal congestion and discharge become severe, over-the-counter medications (such as Afrin, Neo-Synephrine, and Dristan) are useful for a short time. These sprays work by constricting your engorged blood vessels and subsequently shrinking the swollen nasal mucosal tissues, thereby allowing greater movement of air through your nasal passages.

Their immediate effectiveness in controlling your hay fever symptoms might tempt you to continue their use over prolonged periods. But, solving one problem can sometimes create another. If these sprays are used for more than two or three days consecutively, you cannot expect the same nasal relief that you had initially. The nasal tissues become tolerant to the medication and may actually "rebel" by growing more swollen and red, evolving into a serious condition known as *rhinitis medicamentosa.* Your nasal passages will become sore and remain obstructed. The early stage of this *rebound* phenomenon can clear up if you stop using your decongestant nasal spray immediately. A nonmedicated saline spray (Salinex, Ayr, Ocean Mist) will help soothe and moisturize the inflamed areas. In contrast, the prescription nasal sprays, Nasalcrom and steroid inhalers, do not cause this type of rebound nasal congestion. Treatment with oral steroids is often necessary if your condition is severe and has been long-standing.

WHAT IS THE BEST MEDICINE FOR HAY FEVER?

The best medicine for the first-line treatment of your hay fever is a balanced antihistamine/decongestant combination.

The antihistamine in the combination blocks the principal chemical messenger or mediator (histamine) released by your mast cells and prevents continuation of the allergic response. Other mediators, such as the newly understood leukotrienes, also cause nasal congestion and are not blocked effectively by most antihistamines. Thus, even with the newer antihistamines, allergy symptoms may persist. These newer antihistamines, such as Seldane, Hismanal, and Claritin, have an added anti-inflammatory effect and should provide more complete relief of your nasal symptoms. This new generation of antihistamines have the added advantage of being nonsedating at the doses usually prescribed. They are also generally free of a bothersome antihistamine side effect, that of dryness of the mouth, nose, sinus, and other mucous membranes.

The decongestant of the combination directly constricts your blood vessels and helps to reverse your allergic symptoms, reducing the redness and itching of your eyes as well as the congestion that causes swelling.

The best results occur when antihistamines and, as needed, decongestants are taken regularly during the pollen season. Ideally, the antihistamine should be started before you are exposed to allergens and should be continued daily throughout the season. Waiting for nasal congestion to occur results in an uphill battle for your antihistamine. Treatment is now easier because the recommended dose of the newest medicines is once or twice a day, depending on the brand.

HOW DO I CHOOSE FROM THE HUNDREDS OF ALLERGY MEDICATIONS AT WALGREENS?

For your mild, occasional hay fever symptoms or, when on vacation, you find you have forgotten your medication, you can

ANTIHISTAMINE CLASSES: EXAMPLES OF BRANDS

Brand name	Antihistamine	Decongestant	Type*
Alkylamines			
Chlor-Trimeton	Chlorpheniramine maleate, 4, 8, 12 mg		OTC
Actifed	Triprolidine HCL, 2.5 mg	Pseudoephedrine HCL, 60 mg	OTC
Drixoral	Dexbrompheniramine maleate, 6 mg	Pseudoephedrine sulfate, 120 mg	OTC
Rynatan	Chlorpheniramine tannate, 8 mg pyrilamine tannate, 25 mg	Phenylephrine tannate, 25 mg	OTC & Rx
Ethanolamines			
Benadryl	Benadryl 25 mg (OTC), 50 mg (Rx)	Diphenhydramine HCL	OTC & Rx
Tavist-1 (OTC), syrup (Rx)	Clemastine		OTC
Tavist-D	Clemastine 1 mg	Phenylpropanol-amine 75 mg	OTC
Ethylenediamines			
PBZ	Tripelennamine HCL		Rx
Piperazines			
Atarax	Hydroxyzine HCL, 10, 25, 50, 100 mg		Rx
Others			
Seldane	Terfenadine, 60 mg		Rx
Trinalin	Azatadine maleate, 1 mg	Pseudoephedrine sulfate, 120 mg	Rx
Hismanal	Astemizole, 10 mg		Rx
Claritin	Loratadine, 10 mg		Rx

*OTC indicates that the drug is available over-the-counter. Rx indicates that it is available by prescription only.

generally select an effective over-the-counter medication. There are common basic ingredients that you should look for in these many preparations (*see* box).

For nasal congestion, choose a preparation with pseudoephedrine (Sudafed 30 mg, 60 mg) or phenylpropanolamine (12.5 mg, 25 mg) and use the lower dose if you have a tendency toward high blood pressure or if you find yourself becoming irritable. You may consider limited use (no more than two to three days) of a decongestant nasal spray with oxymetazoline (Afrin), phenylephrine (Neo-Synephrine), or xylometazoline (Otrivin). These decongestant nasal sprays are quite helpful before flying, and for nasal and sinus infections.

To treat frequent sneezing and reduce allergy-caused clear nasal discharges, choose a preparation containing such antihistamines as chlorpheniramine (2 to 4 mg), tripolidine (2.5 mg), clemastine (Tavist, 1 mg scored). Again, the lower dose should be chosen or the scored tablet should be divided in half. Diphenhydramine (Benadryl) is good for hives, but it is very sedating and drying. By the way, this same diphenhydramine is the ingredient of almost all over-the-counter sleeping aids.

Choose only the medicinal ingredients you need to treat your hay fever. A combination preparation is often appropriate. Try to avoid those medicines with excessive doses of the compounds you need and those with such unnecessary ingredients as acetaminophen (Tylenol), acetylsalicylic acid (aspirin), caffeine, and dextromethorphan. Aspirin-containing combinations are usually not necessary, and may well be hazardous because aspirin can trigger asthma in certain allergic individuals.

Take only what you need to relieve your symptoms. Excessive use of antihistamines can dry secretions, predisposing and even leading to sinus infections. Sustained-release preparations are convenient, but be sure to look at the ingredients and don't take a time-release medicine if your symptoms are limited only to the early morning. For coughing, guaifenesin and dextromethorphan syrups offer relief, but, again, avoid a potpourri of ingredients.

Some people cannot take a classic or first-generation antihistamine because of the drowsiness and dryness of the mouth they produce, whereas others cannot tolerate a decongestant because of the irritability, headaches, dizziness, or difficulty with high blood pressure they cause. Hypertensive reactions, seizures, and brain hemorrhage have been reported with the common decongestant phenylpropanolamine, which is also an ingredient of diet pills. Other side effects of the antihistamines and decongestants include difficulty with urination in men and/or impotence, aggravation of glaucoma, and decreased production of milk in a nursing mother. Additionally, a type of antidepressant known as an MAO inhibitor should not be taken concurrently with decongestants or tyramine-containing foods such as cheese. This combination can lead to dangerous elevations of the blood pressure. The combination of caffeine and decongestants may speed you up, sometimes producing tremors and even palpitations, and should be avoided. Patients with diabetes, heart disease, or thyroid disease should use decongestants only after consulting their physicians. To sum up, some over-the-counter preparations are effective—antihistamines for runny nose and decongestants for stuffy nose—but these should be used judiciously, and only after careful study of their ingredients and your personal medical circumstances.

The new antihistamines, like the old antihistamines, are also not free of potential problems. A dangerous and sometimes lethal drug interaction has been found: Thus, if you are taking Seldane or Hismanal, you should not take erythromycin and related antibiotics, nor the oral antifungal medications Nizoral (ketoconazole), Sporanox (itraconazole), and possibly Diflucan (fluconazole). These drugs interfere with the metabolism (breakdown) and excretion of the antihistamines in the liver. This causes a buildup of the unmetabolized antihistamines in the blood and these high blood levels in turn are toxic to the heart and cause abnormal heart rhythms and electrocardiogram changes. Also, beware of trouble if you have liver disease. New antihistamines, such as Claritin, will have to be evaluated. Seldane is not prescribed for nursing mothers because it is associated with poor weight gain in puppies.

When hay fever symptoms are severe, you may benefit from one of the newer steroid nasal sprays (Nasalide, Beconase, Vancenase). Your physician may also prescribe prednisone for a short time. Nasalcrom helps some patients by preventing histamine release from nasal mast cells and is best used before you are exposed to grass, ragweed, or your mother-in-law's cat. Ipratropium nasal spray can also be effective. You may need these medications in conjunction with allergy shots to give yourself maximum relief.

Are There Any Stronger Medications Available for Hay Fever?

Recent advances in allergy medication include the steroid nasal sprays: Beconase, Vancenase, Nasalide, and Nasacort. These steroid sprays are very effective for the relief not only of nasal congestion, but also of sneezing, itching, and runny nose. They are anti-inflammatory in their action and thus prevent emergence of the full effects of the allergic hay fever reaction. And they are very effective, especially during the peak hay fever season when antihistamines may fail. These nasal steroids must be distinguished from over-the-counter decongestant nasal sprays. Their regular use is essential and you should expect to wait several days for relief. Whereas the over-the-counter sprays can be habit forming, the steroid sprays are not. Your choice of brand depends greatly on personal preference. Some patients prefer dry aerosols, while others prefer the aqueous, water-based sprays. A potential problem is nosebleeds. This can be lessened by aiming the spray away from the septum and not putting the applicator deep into the nose. If nosebleeds are a problem coat the nasal septum with a small amount of petroleum jelly before using the spray. Though the sprays can be employed for an extended period of time, they should always be used at the lowest dose possible, especially when applied on a year-round basis. Because there is a small but definite absorption of these topical steroids, which can produce changes throughout the body, they should be used sparingly in children. Of course, their use can be minimized by good environmental control and, when necessary, by allergy injections.

An exceedingly safe alternative is cromolyn sodium (Nasalcrom). It does not help as many patients as the steroids, but when it works it is wonderful. Unfortunately, it functions only when taken preventively, usually four times a day. It is an anti-inflammatory medication that is not a steroid.

What Is the Best Medicine for My Eyes?

Your eyes are a ready target for airborne allergens—especially pollens and animal danders. Shelter yourself as soon as symptoms start. Cold compresses and eye rinses such as Artificial Tears can be very helpful. Depending on your preference and response, oral antihistamine–decongestant medications and/or eyedrops may be used. Over-the-counter Visine or Murine may temporarily relieve your problem, but more effective prescription eyedrops (Naphcon-A, Vasocon-A, and Livostin), may be preferable. Sometimes the preservatives in the eyedrops may be irritating. Like nasal sprays, frequent use can result in rebound and the drops become habit forming. Acular (ketorolac) and Alomide (lodoxamine) are nonsteroidal anti-inflammatory eyedrops that can relieve itching and inflammation of the eyes.

Cromolyn 4% eyedrops are very useful when used on a regular basis to prevent allergic eye symptoms. These are especially recommended for long-term symptoms; they are safe and can also help you break the habit of excessive use of irritating decongestant solutions. Currently, a pharmacist will have to compound cromolyn eyedrops on your physician's order. They must be used four to six times a day prior to your exposure to the allergens whose effects you have to avoid. In England, a new preventive compound called nedocromil is available for the eyes and is expected to be available eventually in the United States. It has already been released here in the asthma formulation, Tilade.

Corticosteroid eyedrops, oral prednisone, or injectable steroids should be used only in the most severe and unresponsive situations. Close medical supervision is necessary because of possible complications with glaucoma, or with herpes and other eye infections. Never use last year's leftover prescription this year.

CAN I TAKE HAY FEVER MEDICATIONS FOR A LONG TIME?

Yes. The antihistamines and decongestants prescribed for your hay fever may be taken for many years. Possible side effects, however, should be monitored. These may occur even when the duration of treatment is only a few days. Since some tolerance to antihistamines often develops, switching to a different class of these compounds may renew effectiveness when yours loses its ability to relieve your symptoms.

CAN SOME DENTAL PROBLEMS BE CAUSED BY ALLERGIES?

Children who are mouth breathers because of allergic rhinitis may develop facial and dental deformities associated with underdevelopment of the mid-face. They often develop elongated faces and high-arch palates, and suffer a greater incidence of dental crossbites and overbites that require orthodontic treatment. Persistent congestion, teeth grinding, and snoring (with short periods of no breathing, called sleep apnea) are an indication of enlarged adenoids. Be sure to report these symptoms to your pediatrician when you first notice them. Efforts should be made to correct the cause of chronic mouth breathing during the developing childhood years.

CAN HAY FEVER LEAD TO ASTHMA?

Yes. When you have severe hay fever with both nasal and eye symptoms you may well start wheezing. The allergic reaction causing hay fever can indeed extend to the lungs, causing inflammation with constriction of your bronchioles and a wheezing sound on expiration. The wheezing sometimes starts when your nasal and eye symptoms become very severe. At other times, the hay fever lessens and your asthma becomes the main allergic manifestation. This post-seasonal bronchial hyperreactivity then can become a self-perpetuating, ongoing wheeze. Desensitization (allergy shots) has been helpful in preventing this asthmatic reaction in some people. Nevertheless, allergy shots for hay fever will not prevent the later development of genetically inherited, nonallergic asthma. Environmental control—focused on such measures as the removal of carpets and mattress encasings to eliminate dust mites, as well as keeping animals out of the house—is necessary if you, your child, or anyone in your household suffers from asthma. These preventive measures are truly cost effective, as well as the best treatment for asthma—far more important than expensive new medications and allergy shots.

Finally, the relationship of asthma and hay fever has been an interesting unresolved question in medical research. About 40% of hay fever patients will demonstrate some asthmatic changes during pulmonary function testing after such vigorous exercise as running—even though they have no obvious symptoms of clinical asthma. However, only 5% of children with hay fever go on to develop bronchial asthma.

WHAT ABOUT CHRISTMAS TREES?

Christmas trees cause allergic symptoms in many people. The most common sources of difficulty are the airborne pollens and molds that are naturally to be found in the trees, and that remain there after they have been cut down and stored. A person who is sensitive to these pollens and molds will come into close contact with them when a large, moist tree comes into the home. The heat of the house helps to release these inhalant substances into the closed indoor environment, and thus a family recreates, for a few weeks in December, a specific allergy-inducing pollen or mold season.

Studies have indicated that a chemical, terpene, is released by the tree itself. This substance directly causes allergy-like symptoms—nasal congestion, discharge, and wheezing—in a sensitive individual. People who switch to artificial Christmas trees no longer suffer the problem and remain well enough to enjoy the holiday season, at least as long as they clean the tree of dust each year before use.

DO I HAVE "SINUS"?

Because of fullness in the nasal area, the term "sinus" is frequently used to describe the nasal stuffiness associated with hay fever by its sufferers. Your sinuses are cavities with openings to the nasal passages and are lined with membranes similar to those in the nose. The main sinuses are located above your eyes (frontal), between your eyes (ethmoid), and behind your cheek bones (maxillary).

The medical term sinusitis refers to inflammation or infection of the sinuses. When your sinus openings are blocked by the swollen allergic nasal membranes, pressure changes occur and are probably the cause of most recurrent sinus headaches. The

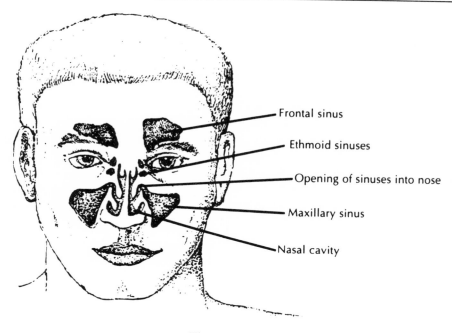

The sinuses.

often intense pain can be relieved by reducing the swelling of the membranes. Even in children, many patients with chronic allergic nasal symptoms may develop sinus infections.

When your sinus openings are blocked and mucus is present, ideal conditions for infection with bacteria are created. Bacterial growth causes the development of pus which, in turn, pushes against the walls of the clogged sinuses, causing pain. Bacterial infections of your sinuses require prompt medical attention.

This pain is most severe over your sinuses—under the eyes, "behind" the eyes, and in the forehead over the eyes. The pain may also radiate to the back of the head. Yellow or green pus may discharge from your nose or drip into the back of your throat, causing irritation and cough. If your infection goes untreated the sinus can rupture, enabling bacteria and pus to enter the brain, a rare but serious and potentially fatal complication.

Swimming and scuba diving should be avoided if you have an acute sinus infection. Among frequent fliers the dry, contaminated air, together with the rapid pressure changes common in the cabin, contribute to recurrent sinusitis.

HOW DO YOU DIAGNOSE AND TREAT SINUSITIS?

Sinusitis is usually diagnosed clinically on the basis of history and physical examination. If you are fortunate enough to clear up your sinus infection with antibiotics alone, there is no problem. However, persistent or recurrent sinus symptoms present a difficult situation. Chronic headaches, fatigue, and the loss of your sense of smell need evaluation. Failure to respond to the necessary 2–3 week course of antibiotics, decongestants, expectorants, and cortisone nasal sprays indicates the need for further investigation and more aggressive treatment. Sinus X-rays have recently been superceded by a helpful new technology—the CT scan, a sophisticated X-ray that provides an accurate, precise, almost three-dimensional look at the sinus cavities. Until now we could not see the ethmoid sinuses located behind the nose and between the eyes, where most chronic sinus infections lurk. The CT scan is a fast, safe and painless, though rather expensive, procedure.

It is important to drain your infected sinuses. Thinning and liquefying the secretions can be helpful. High-dose guaifenesin (Fenesin, Humibid) along with combinations of guaifenesin and decongestants, in addition to steam inhalation and nasal irrigation with saline, are all effective. A very short course of oral steroids (prednisone) is sometimes necessary in resistant cases.

Choosing the preferred antibiotic is difficult because of the emergence of germs resistant to many antibiotics. Your doctor should choose the one for you that has the fewest side effects. Generally, erythromycin and plain penicillin are not helpful. Sometimes the combination of two antibiotics may even be necessary! During the winter cold season, long-term, daily preventive antibiotic treatment is often helpful.

Ear, nose, and throat specialists have also developed a new endoscopic surgical procedure using a fiberoptic device that is inserted directly into the nose. The device contains tiny instruments that are manuevered under direct visualization to remove swollen, infected, diseased mucosal linings from the sinuses.

Polyps can also be removed and the sinus openings enlarged. Although this surgery has been very helpful to many, the conditions it treats often recur and it is therefore always necessary to address the causative allergic, irritant, or infective factors.

CAN SINUSITIS CAUSE ASTHMA?

There is a high association of chronic sinusitis with exacerbations of asthma. It is not known for sure that sinusitis causes asthma, but when sinusitis is controlled, asthma is frequently lessened. This relationship is sometimes called the sinopulmonary reflex. Chronic sinusitis is often a hidden trigger for asthma (cough and wheeze). The appropriate use of CT scans and endoscopic surgery to reduce or eliminate sinusitis has benefited many asthma patients.

WHY DO MY EARS HURT, CRACKLE, AND POP?

The eustachian tube connects your middle ear (behind the ear drum) to the back of your nasal–throat area. Normally this tube allows adjustment of the pressure in your ears—for example, at high altitudes or diving. If you suffer allergies, your eustachian tubes can become swollen and then malfunction. This leads to a sensation of pressure in your ears with pain, popping, and crackling. Fluid may also accumulate in your middle ear, leading to hearing loss with consequential school difficulties, and to the possible occurrence of infections requiring antibiotics. This condition frequently responds to decongestants if treated early, but if the fluid remains in the eustachian tube for a prolonged time, it becomes sticky (glue ear) and surgical treatment may be necessary. Placement of tubes in your eardrums, and sometimes removal of enlarged adenoids, allows your eustachian tube to function normally. Sometimes persistent fluid will clear after a short-term course of prednisone and antibiotics.

COULD MY HEADACHES BE CAUSED BY TMJ?

Yes. A totally nonallergic cause of headache and ear pain is "temporomandibular joint syndrome" (TMJ), alternately called temporomandibular joint dysfunction. This is a painful inflammation of the joint connecting your jaw or mandible to the temporal bone of your skull—right in front of your ear. TMJ often produces pain, difficulty in opening the mouth, a clicking sensation in the jaw, pain with chewing, headaches, neckaches, and dental pain. Since more than 50% of the population experiences occasional clicking when the jaw is moved, it is also important to evaluate the range of motion of your jaw. Thus, you should be able to open your mouth at least one and one-half inches (40 millimeters) and you should be able to move your jaw from side to side without difficulty. Patients are often convinced that the pain from their TMJ originates in the ears and that their ears are filled with fluid. Examination of the ears reveals normal eardrums even as pressure on the joint, especially when opening the jaw, can elicit symptoms. Mild or intermittent cases respond very well to the over-the-counter anti-inflammatory drug ibuprofen and a soft diet. If this doesn't work, an evaluation by a dentist knowledgeable in TMJ syndrome is necessary.

WHAT IS VASOMOTOR RHINITIS?

Vasomotor rhinitis is a common condition frequently confused with allergy. The suspected diagnosis emerges from medical history taking and is confirmed when allergy skin tests prove negative or do not correlate with the appearance of symptoms. Rhinitis means inflammation of the nose. Basically, your nasal mucosa or lining can react to the environment in two ways: they can secrete clear mucus (a runny nose) or they can become swollen (a stuffy nose). In some, these allergy-like symptoms are a reaction to such physical factors as temperature change, air pollution, humidity change, or odors (perfumes). Emotions may play a role, and even sunshine may trigger a sneezing reflex. Vasomotor refers to the motor nerves that control the engorgement or constriction of the blood vessels and regulate the edema (swelling) and the clear watery secretion of the mucous membranes. Some vasomotor rhinitis sufferers also experience eye itching, irritation, and watering.

One function of your nose is to warm and humidify the air you breathe. Inspired air passes over bony structures in your nose covered with moist mucous membranes called turbinates. Normally your turbinates swell and contract, alternating left to right. Lying down causes the dependent turbinate to swell so that one side of your nose becomes partially or completely blocked. Persistently swollen turbinates can completely block your nose. You should suspect vasomotor rhinitis if you develop a stuffy, runny nose and sneezing when you get out of the shower on a cold morning, come indoors from a cold environment, or go outdoors on a hot and smoggy, or a cold and foggy, day. Often, vasomotor and allergic rhinitis occur together.

Vasomotor rhinitis sufferers must rely on medications when symptoms are severe and trigger factors cannot be avoided. Ordinary over-the-counter decongestant sprays can temporarily shrink the membranes of your nose, but invariably create a vicious cycle of rebound as the turbinate swellings worsen with continued use, thus becoming habit forming. Intranasal cortisone sprays, including Beconase, Vancenase, Nasacort, and Nasalide, are helpful and safe when used as directed by your physician. Topical cortisones have a much slower onset of action over several days, but rebound does not occur. Overuse or improper use of steroids can, unfortunately, lead to nosebleeds. Periodic examination of your nose is necessary. Care should be taken not to traumatize your nasal septum with the steroid applicator. Some patients obtain relief by using oral decongestants, such as pseudoephedrine (Sudafed) or phenylpropanolamine, which are available under many brand names. Decongestants taken by mouth can also cause rebound and exacerbate existing high blood pressure. Ipratropium nasal spray (Atrovent) may also provide relief. Vigorous aerobic exercise, such as running or circuit weight training, may give temporary, nonmedication relief by releasing your own epinephrine (adrenalin).

DOES A DEVIATED SEPTUM COMPLICATE ALLERGY?

The bone that divides your nose into the right and left sides— the septum—is often closer to one side, narrowing that opening. You may be born with a significantly deviated septum, or the deviation may result from injury. When your nasal membranes are swollen from allergy, the obstruction may become more severe, completely blocking one side of the nose. The turbinate on the wider side may then swell, causing bothersome, persistent nasal obstruction. Your physician may be able to diagnose a septal deviation by a simple examination of the nose, but sometimes a CT scan or an endoscopic examination is necessary to determine the exact degree of deviation. This is a complicated procedure that requires experience and expertise. Surgery can relieve the bothersome obstruction when the condition is severe.

IS NASAL ENDOSCOPY HELPFUL?

Nasal endoscopy allows your physician to enter the nasal and sinus cavities with a fiberoptic instrument and thus to see more:

- Hidden polyps
- The sinus openings themselves
- Infected secretions
- Foreign bodies, such as tiny toys
- Tumors
- The back of the nasal septum
- The adenoid tissue
- Opening of the eustachian tube
- The larynx, or voice box

With local anesthetics this office procedure causes minimal discomfort while giving valuable information.

WHAT ABOUT KIDS WHO PUT THINGS IN THEIR NOSES?

Small toys and sometimes pieces of food are often found in the nostrils of a child producing yellowish or green secretions and a congestion limited to one side of the nose. This sometimes masquerades as an allergy, at least until a careful examination reveals otherwise

WHERE DO NASAL POLYPS ORIGINATE?

Polyps originate in the sinuses. They are formed when a surface of the membrane becomes loaded with fluids and swells to accommodate the excess. Portions of this membrane then bulge out, fill the sinuses, and protrude into the nose, frequently blocking the nasal passages.

Nasal polyps are not tumors, and their relation to allergy is disputed. There is a high incidence of asthma in patients with polyps and, interestingly, severe asthma may be triggered in this class of asthmatics when they take aspirin. In children polyps may indicate cystic fibrosis.

Polyps occasionally disappear, but treatment is usually desirable. The new cortisone nasal sprays should be tried first; but, oral prednisone may be required to shrink the polyps. Surgical removal by the endoscopic technique is often necessary. The treatment of polyps is frustrating because they frequently recur in spite of all measures taken.

3

Asthma

What Is Happening in My Chest?
Is Asthma Always Allergic?
Why Do I Wheeze Four Hours Later?
I Wheeze All the Time. How Can I Be Allergic to My Dog?
Is It Important to Find Out Whether My Asthma Is Caused
    by Allergies?
Can Asthma Be Caused by Mold Allergies?
Will Allergy Shots Help My Asthma?
Is Asthma Hereditary?
Why Asthma at My Age?
Why Do I Wake Up Wheezing?
What Else Can Cause Wheezing?
How Would a Chest X-Ray Help?
Why Does My Child Need a Sweat Test for Cystic Fibrosis?
Does Coughing Trigger Asthma?
Is Asthma Like Emphysema?
What About Infections and Antibiotics?
How About Flu Vaccine?
Can an Infection Actually Lead to the Onset of Asthma?
Is Asthma Emotionally Triggered?
Is Biofeedback Helpful?
Can My Job Make My Asthma Worse?
Can Asthma Be Caused by Allergy to Tobacco Smoke?
What Is the Best Way to Stop Smoking?
What About Cigaret Smoking and Marijuana?
Can Stoves and Fireplaces Be a Problem?
Can a Single Exposure to an Irritating Gas or Smoke Give Me Asthma
    for Years?
What About Sulfite Preservatives?
What Is the Chinese Restaurant Syndrome?

3 ASTHMA

Can I Drink Alcohol?
Sex?
Is Scuba Diving Compatible with Asthma?
Should I Get Pregnant?
Can I Take Asthma Medications If I Am Pregnant?
Should I Stop My Asthma Medications If I Am Pregnant?
Is Asthma Contagious?
What Is the Best Medicine for Asthma?
What Are Beta Agonists?
What About the Drug That Prevents Wheezing?
Are Steroids Dangerous?
Will the Steroids I Take for Asthma and Allergy Give Me Great Muscles?
Can There Be Complications with Chickenpox When I Am Taking Steroids?
Why Don't My Inhaled Steroids Work?
Do I Need a Peak Flow Meter?
How Can I Determine My Personal Best Peak Flow Value?
What Is an Asthma Control Plan?
What Should I Expect in the Emergency Room?
Which Drugs Must I Avoid If I Have Asthma?
May I Play Sports?
What About Backpacking?
Should I Go to Asthma Camp?
Can I Die from Asthma?
Should I Move?
Can Asthma Be Cured?

What Is Happening in My Chest?

Bronchial asthma is, as the name implies, a disease affecting the bronchial tubes. Asthma is an inflammation of the lining of your bronchial tubes. Air enters the chest through the trachea, commonly called the "windpipe." The trachea then divides into the right and left mainstem bronchi. These tubes themselves divide again and again to form many hundreds of tiny bronchial tubes or bronchioles. Strands of muscles encircle the bronchial tubes.

In the lining of the bronchial tubes there are mucus-producing cells, the goblet cells, which are covered with tiny, hairlike fibers called cilia. The mucus produced by the goblet cells traps invasive particles and substances, and with a beating motion, the cilia move the mucus and its trapped materials up from the bronchial tubes through the trachea. In this way the bronchial tubes clean themselves.

During an episode of asthma your bronchial muscles involuntarily contract, constricting the inflamed bronchial tubes. The inflammation itself is caused by the action of your white blood cells, such as eosinophils and neutrophils, that enter the bronchial walls by a process of transmigration through the blood vessel walls. The eosinophils contain and release a potent toxic substance, major basic protein, that causes most of the damage in your asthma by stimulating the mast cells to release those chemicals or mediators that initiate your lung's inflammation. Major basic protein also directly causes your bronchial tubes to become irritable and twitchy, and by doing so, causes your goblet cells to produce very large amounts of sticky mucus (phlegm). If your asthma continues unchecked, then the bronchial walls become swollen and inflamed and further narrowing of your airways occurs.

When your chest expands during inhalation, air enters your bronchial tubes on its way down to the tiny breathing sacs (alveoli) at the ends of the tubes. When you, the asthmatic, exhale, these bronchial tubes become even smaller and air is trapped in your lungs. Air passing through these narrowed tubes as you breathe in and out creates a musical sound—wheezing—

ASTHMA

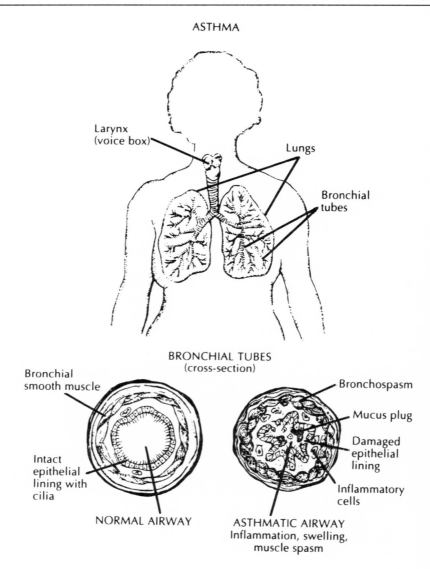

Asthma.

and a sensation of tightness in your chest. The mucus forms sticky plugs that further narrow some of your air passages, and close others completely. When air cannot move in and out, you begin to feel short of breath, or dyspneic, and your blood flows through the walls of the alveoli without picking up the needed oxygen or giving off your excess carbon dioxide.

Is Asthma Always Allergic?

This is an important question and deserves some discussion. If you find a new home for your cat and you stop wheezing, do you still have asthma? The answer is yes. Anyone who wheezes has bronchial tubes that are more irritable than those of the non-asthmatic's lungs, and thus is susceptible to episodes of asthma.

If you wheeze only because of your specific allergy, removal of the allergen (in this case, your cat) will eliminate your asthma. Years later, however, a visit to your aunt who has a cat can once again trigger an episode.

At the other end of the spectrum there is a population of asthmatics with no allergic cause. Within this group there is a wide range of severity. Some people have only occasional flareups, whereas others wheeze all the time and need constant medication. We find our most severe patients with life-threatening asthma in this latter group. The important trigger factors here include infections, air pollution, tobacco smoke, occupational exposures, sulfite preservatives, cold air, exercise, emotional upset, and in some patients aspirin and aspirin-related drugs such as ibuprofen (Advil).

Most likely your asthma has an allergic component. Specific allergens, in addition to any other irritating trigger factors in your environment, will cause an episode of wheezing. These allergens may be hidden, and may include dust mites, molds, and foods. Generally, allergy plays a role in most childhood asthma and in a significant percentage of adult asthma. Some asthma—particularly those cases that start in later life—may not be at all associated with allergy, and are historically called intrinsic asthma.

Why Do I Wheeze Four Hours Later?

After exposure to allergens at home or at work, your asthma may flare up only some four to eight hours later. This is known as late-phase reaction asthma. It is caused by an inflammation of your bronchial tubes initiated by the allergic reaction, an inflammation that then progresses in the absence of any further allergen exposure. Your late-phase reaction and its consequent asthma can last up to five days!

Examples of the process may be seen in the following cases: While visiting a friend with a cat, you notice some nasal congestion and mild wheezing. You use your asthma inhaler (albuterol, salmeterol, etc.) with good relief only to have the asthma recur long after you get home. Similarly, the veterinary assistant may be fine at work, only to have asthma trouble at home on the weekends. The best treatment in either case is the regular use of inhaled anti-inflammatories such as steroids, Intal (cromolyn), or Tilade (nedocromil). For severe, acute reactions, injected or oral steroids may be necessary.

I Wheeze All the Time. How Can I Be Allergic to My Dog?

You have a dog, but you continue to wheeze while you are at work or away for the weekend. You come home to the dog, and the wheezing is no more severe. Nevertheless, the dog may still be the cause. Chronic, late-phase reaction or wheezing explains this phenomenon. If you were able to stay away from the dog for weeks at a time, then you might see that the asthma would clear, and only flare again when you returned home. A positive skin test—prick test, and often a necessary intradermal test if the prick test proves negative—can confirm the diagnosis of allergy to your own dog. Unfortunately, you will now need to remove the dog from your home. And since significant animal dander may persist for up to six months after the pet is removed, an intense cleaning and scrubbing effort must be mounted.

Is It Important to Find Out Whether My Asthma Is Caused by Allergies?

Consultation with an allergist is imperative for anyone with asthma. If you can identify a specific allergic component to your asthma, then you can possibly remove or treat the cause. Why just keep taking more medicine? Conversely, why should you remove your cat and endure the aggravation of a rigorous dust control program if you are not allergic?

CAN ASTHMA BE CAUSED BY MOLD ALLERGIES?

One of the most compelling reasons for an allergy evaluation is to diagnose a severe asthmatic condition related to mold allergy—*allergic bronchopulmonary aspergillosis*. This is a severe allergic condition that, if untreated, can permanently damage your lungs and the diagnosis is occasionally missed. It is somewhat more prevalent in colder wet climates, but should always be considered in cases of difficult to control asthma.

Your workup begins with a carefully taken allergy and medical history. Your allergy skin testing will include Aspergillus, a commonly found airborne mold spore. If the skin test is positive, the workup proceeds with a chest X-ray or CT scan. Laboratory studies are necessary for confirmation of the diagnosis, and characteristic abnormalities include very high levels of specific and total IgE antibodies, and elevated blood eosinophils. The condition fortunately responds well to adequate treatment with prednisone, together with other asthma medications. Prevention consists of eliminations and avoidance of exposure to mold spores.

Beware of such moldy environments as:

- Damp basements
- Air conditioning systems
- Home or office renovation
- Grain storage bins

If you live in a moldy house; despite all control measures, a move may be necessary.

WILL ALLERGY SHOTS HELP MY ASTHMA?

Allergy shots (immunotherapy) can be helpful to many whose asthma is caused by allergy to pollens, house dust mites, animal danders, and molds. Such shots work by treating the allergy that triggers your asthma rather than the asthma itself, and research has strongly confirmed that immunotherapy can indeed substantially improve such asthma. Of course, the best treatment for animal allergies is the permanent removal of your pet from the house.

Allergy shots have helped many of the authors' asthmatic patients tolerate the spring and summer pollen seasons. And most are now also able to visit the homes of friends and relatives who have cats and dogs.

If your allergy is controlled by immunotherapy shots or by the avoidance of the allergen, then it is less likely that upper respiratory infections or airborne irritants will exacerbate an episode of asthma.

Is Asthma Hereditary?

The tendency toward asthma may be inherited, and many asthmatics have relatives with asthma. If both your parents have asthma, then the chance is 70% that you will develop asthma; if one of your parents is affected, then the chance is 40%. Environmental and developmental factors are also important. The inheritance of asthma is said to be *polygenic*, meaning that many gene units are involved and must be present in just the right combination for your asthma to develop.

Why Asthma at My Age?

Asthma may strike at *any* age. The onset of asthma frequently occurs in infancy and most childhood asthma starts by the time of the first grade. The disease is so prevalent among school age children in this country that an estimated ten million school days a year are missed because of asthma attacks. It is also the number one reason children are admitted to the hospital. Before puberty, boys have more trouble with asthma than girls, but by puberty many boys outgrow their asthma. On the other hand, after puberty women have more trouble with asthma. A new pet in the house might trigger asthma in a teenager. Commonly without warning and sometimes without allergic cause, asthma develops in the menopausal years. Asthma that develops in childhood may subside only to reappear in later life. Additionally, asthma may occur in an adult who previously had eczema or hay fever in childhood.

Children with mild asthma have a better chance of outgrowing their problem, and generally do so by puberty. If significant asthma persists into the teenage years, it is likely to be lifelong; but even so, as many as 50% of these 14-year-olds can expect to have less trouble later on.

WHY DO I WAKE UP WHEEZING?

Allergists should work at night! After all, dust mites live on the mattresses and under the beds of their patients, so that allergen exposure can be greater at night. Moreover, your bronchial tubes are more reactive since cortisol and adrenalin levels decline nightly with your body's natural circadian (daily) rhythm. It is very important to control your nocturnal asthma since this is when most life-threatening episodes occur.

There are some conditions that are neither wheezing nor asthma, but the symptoms are sometimes confused with those of asthma. These are sounds that come from the larynx (voice box) or the nose. One such interesting condition is called paradoxical vocal cord dysfunction. When someone with this condition inhales, instead of opening, the vocal cords close and cause a wheezing or stridorous noise. Remember, asthmatics wheeze only when they exhale. The treatment for this distressing condition is relaxation. In another condition, partial obstruction of the nasal passages sometimes produces a whistle-like sound.

Frequent nocturnal asthma requires an increase in your inhaled steroids; Proventil Repetabs and Volmax may be helpful, as well as long-acting theophylline. The position of your body is also important. Mucus dripping from the sinuses and the nose can trigger wheezing. When some people lie down, stomach acid is refluxed into the esophagus. This then causes irritation (heartburn) and can trigger asthma. The condition is known as gastroesophageal reflux disease (GERD), and those with significant reflux may wheeze even through the day and awaken with heartburn and a sour taste in the mouth. Raising the head of your bed may help, but extra pillows just bend your body and make the situation worse. Obese patients often suffer an increased incidence of reflux, and weight reduction may help. If you fall into either of these categories, don't eat for at least several hours before sleeping. Since gastroesophageal reflux may itself be a serious medical problem, treatment must be individualized.

WHAT ELSE CAN CAUSE WHEEZING?

Besides asthma, wheezing can occur in other medical conditions such as pneumonia and bronchitis. In the young child wheezing may be associated with an anatomical obstruction around the airways (blood vessels, tumor, malformations). Aspiration of food particles, such as peanuts, hot dogs, or small toy parts, into the windpipe can also cause wheezing.

In the young child with persistent cough, wheeze, and sometimes failure to thrive, cystic fibrosis should be considered. In adults, there may be a localized pulmonary infection or a tumor—especially in smokers. Congestive heart failure can also be characterized by wheezing, especially at night or after exercise.

HOW WOULD A CHEST X-RAY HELP?

A chest X-ray is used primarily to help rule out other conditions that may be clinically confused with asthma. These include:

- A tiny toy accidentally swallowed and trapped in the bronchi of a toddler
- Pneumonia
- A tumor
- A congenital vascular condition in an infant (with barium swallow)
- Heart failure

A chest X-ray also helps identify a complication of asthma called pneumothorax (ruptured lung) and scars from previous lung infections including tuberculosis, valley fever (California and Arizona), and histoplasmosis (midwest).

WHY DOES MY CHILD NEED A SWEAT TEST FOR CYSTIC FIBROSIS?

Cystic fibrosis can initially present with asthma symptoms and repeated pneumonias. This is the most common inherited disease of white children and is carried on the chromosome 7.

African-Americans can also have cystic fibrosis, but the incidence is about ten times less frequent. Early diagnosis is very important for starting appropriate medical management of this serious genetic condition.

DOES COUGHING TRIGGER ASTHMA?

Many asthmatics say, "If I could only stop coughing, I wouldn't wheeze." They are sometimes correct: postnasal drip and excess mucus irritate the throat or trachea and the coughing can trigger the spasms of asthma. Conversely, a cough is frequently the first and only sign of asthma itself. This is true in both children and adults.

Coughing and wheezing are caused by the same mechanism—inflammation and bronchospasm. When your asthma's wheezing or inflammation is relieved, your cough will also subside. Pulmonary function testing is an important diagnostic tool. A therapeutic trial with bronchodilators and such anti-inflammatories as cromolyn, nedocromil, or inhaled steroids can confirm the diagnosis as well as provide relief. Inhaled *Atrovent* may be particularly helpful if your cough is a major manifestation of irritable airways.

IS ASTHMA LIKE EMPHYSEMA?

Emphysema and asthma are quite dissimilar. Asthma is, by definition, a reversible or controllable disease; that is, with proper treatment normal breathing can be restored, at least temporarily. In emphysema, the alveoli and lung tissue are actually destroyed. When the small bronchial airways are irreversibly damaged (often by smoking), the diagnosis of chronic obstructive pulmonary disease (COPD) is made.

There is also an inherited deficiency of an enzyme known as alpha-1-antitrypsin that causes a form of emphysema together with liver disease. A characteristic chest X-ray pattern shows destruction of the lung tissue at the bases. A blood test can diagnose this condition and treatment may be helpful.

There is currently research interest in the possibility that chronic, long-term, severe, untreated asthma may progress to a condition similar to COPD. For this reason we disagree with the attitude of some parents that their children will "grow out of it" or can "tough it out." You should always consider asthma serious.

There is considerable similarity, however, with respect to the medications used to treat all of these lung diseases. Atrovent is much more helpful in relieving the symptoms of emphysema than it generally is with those of asthma. For exacerbations of emphysema, systemic cortisone or prednisone is essential. Inhaled steroids can stop the accelerated progression in the loss of lung function that emphysema causes. At any stage in the diseases, patients with asthma or emphysema should stop smoking and avoid second-hand smoke. It is never too late to stop smoking!

WHAT ABOUT INFECTIONS AND ANTIBIOTICS?

Infections can cause asthma. Those that affect asthma are such common respiratory adversaries as influenza, the common cold, and sinus infections. People with asthma tend to develop respiratory infections more often than those free of the disease.

Sinus pains, increased nasal congestion, wheezing, chest tightness, an exacerbation of coughing spells with discolored sputum are all symptoms of a respiratory infection, as are the familiar general fatigue, headaches, and fever. You should always be on the alert for these signs, and take every reasonable measure to treat them, and thereby prevent the buildup of an asthma attack.

When possible, you should stay away from people with colds and other respiratory illnesses. Keep in mind that being in crowded places during the fall and winter months exposes you to others' infections. And regular handwashing is critical.

Antibiotics, such as the penicillins, erythromycin, and tetracycline, may or may not be helpful. Do not be misled by thinking that antibiotics will always cure your infections and alleviate your asthma. In fact, only infections that are caused by bacteria need to be treated with antibiotics. Since colds and influenza are caused by viruses, it is unreasonable to take antibiotics for their cure unless your doctor wants you to do so to prevent a bacterial disease from taking advantage of your system's weakness. If you think that an antibiotic is necessary, ask your physician to evaluate the infection and confirm your need for it.

HOW ABOUT FLU VACCINE?

If you have asthma requiring regular followup visits, you should get an annual flu vaccination in the fall. Egg-sensitive individuals should be tested. Additionally, your doctor may recommend Pneumovax, a vaccination for a common type of pneumonia. Antiviral drugs are currently being used for the prevention and treatment of certain types of epidemic flu: Symmetrel and Flumadine.

CAN AN INFECTION ACTUALLY LEAD TO THE ONSET OF ASTHMA?

Yes. In the young child a common viral respiratory infection such as bronchiolitis or croup can trigger the onset of infectious asthma. The flu and other viruses can act in a similar way in older children and adults. With subsequent colds, wheezing is likely to recur, and this may predispose the child to the future development of allergic asthma. Allergenic sensitization, with the development of the child's IgE antibodies during one of these viral infections, may well set the stage for the subsequent development of that child's allergic asthma.

In some adults a lung infection with Chlamydia, a microscopic, nonviral, nonbacterial infection, may trigger asthma.

IS ASTHMA EMOTIONALLY TRIGGERED?

There are certainly some individuals who have observed their asthma worsen when they become angry or excited. In these cases therapy is directed at controlling these emotional upsets, this stress that triggers the asthmatic attack. Most of the time, however, it is difficult to sort out exactly how important emotional stress is in causing asthma. In our experience as physicians, emotions have been exaggerated as a possible cause of asthma attacks, and have often unnecessarily become the primary focus of parental concern. Our view is that emotional stress should be regarded as only one of many possible aggravating factors in asthma, but that such stress must be equally considered and evaluated by a physician.

As with any chronic disease, asthma frequently *causes* stress. It is very important to be aware of this in order to deal with asthma effectively and put it in perspective.

Is Biofeedback Helpful?

Stress can trigger wheezing and wheezing in turn creates stress. This cycle must be broken when you are seeking to get your asthma under control. The various techniques used to break the cycle are collectively called behavior modification, with mindfulness exercises, including yoga, tai chi, and meditation.

If you are able to teach your body to respond appropriately to various stimuli, you may be able to help "switch off" your asthma. The usefulness of such breathing exercises lies in learning to relax and not panic while waiting for your medication to work. Individualized behavior modification can be integrated into the treatment of your asthma. We have seen patients who have, by trial and error, learned how to use these techniques.

Can My Job Make My Asthma Worse?

Obviously, yes, if your environment exposes you to substances to which you are allergic or sensitive (*see* box on opposite page).

If you notice relief from asthma on your days off, you should suspect that the cause of your asthma is work-related. However, be aware that asthmatic symptoms may be delayed in onset and be of long duration, say, over the weekend. You should use a peak flow meter to measure your breathing at home and at work, and monitor changes. Quitting your job may not always be a desirable solution. Taking certain asthma medications before going to work and wearing a face mask or respirator may help. You should encourage your employer to improve ventilation or, if possible, transfer you to another work location where you will not be exposed to the troublesome substance.

IRRITANTS IN THE WORK ENVIRONMENT

Allergic:
- Animals—rats, mice, guinea pigs, rabbits, mice, cats, dogs, and horses (laboratory workers, veterinarians, and jockeys)
- Pollens (gardeners and telephone linemen)
- Dust and molds (janitors and housekeepers)
- Fish (food handlers)
- Latex rubbers (health care workers; meat processors)
- Flour (bakers)
- MDI and TDI–diisocyanates (plastic polyurethane industry)

Nonallergic:
- Soldering flux (electricians)
- Exhaust fumes (auto mechanics)
- Chemical substances (factory workers)
- Sawdust (carpenters)
- Cigaret smoke (bartenders)
- Chalk dust (teachers)

CAN ASTHMA BE CAUSED BY ALLERGY TO TOBACCO SMOKE?

Tobacco smoke is a nonallergic irritant that usually causes more irritation in allergic individuals than in the general population. Moreover, studies have shown higher levels of allergy antibodies (IgE) in smokers, suggesting that smoking itself may exacerbate allergy in the smoker. If you smoke in your home, research has proven that your children or spouse will have significantly more asthma and respiratory infections. It is as if they were smoking a few cigarets a day themselves. Ask for the nonsmoking section whether eating out or flying.

With respect to tobacco itself, a small percentage of asthmatics, especially tobacco workers, have positive skin tests for allergy to tobacco leaf.

WHAT IS THE BEST WAY TO STOP SMOKING?

A disciplined, highly motivated approach is essential. You have to want to seriously stop smoking. Support groups—such as Smokers Anonymous or other groups you might find meeting in

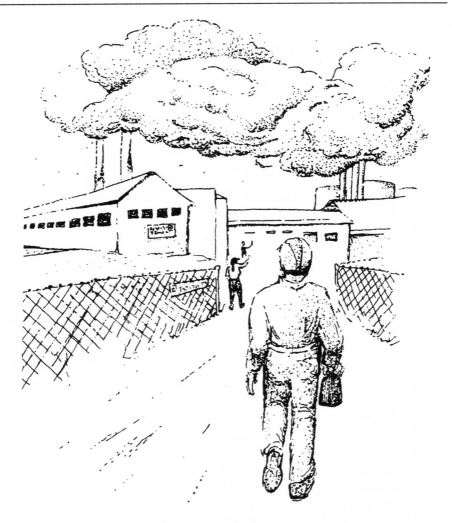

Occupational allergy.

your local hospital, the American Lung Association, or even in the Yellow Pages—can keep you on track. Nicotine patches and nicotine chewing gum (Nicorette) have been used successfully and decrease the craving. It is very important not to smoke when you have the patch on or when you are chewing the nicotine gum; doing so can result in dangerously high levels of nicotine in your system with severe side effects. Another approach is to use clonidine (Catapres), a blood pressure medicine that lessens the symptoms of nicotine withdrawal.

WHAT ABOUT CIGARET SMOKING AND MARIJUANA?

Tobacco smoke is a strong irritant that triggers the bronchospasm of asthma. Asthmatics who smoke often deny the adverse effects of their habit, yet nonsmoking asthmatics report that tobacco smoke is the worst irritant of all. Inhalation of cigaret smoke causes narrowing of your small bronchial tubes and counteracts the effects of your asthma medications. In short, if you have asthma, you and members of your household should not smoke. Sometimes there will be a temporary flareup of cough and wheezing when a person with asthma stops smoking, but this is much less serious than continued exacerbation of your asthma.

The "active" ingredient of marijuana smoke, tetrahydrocannabinol (THC), is actually a mild bronchodilator. As a result, there is a popular misbelief that smoking marijuana is good for asthmatics. Currently available bronchodilating drugs are many times more effective than THC, and avoid the risks of legal consequences. New research shows that the smoke of one "joint" is 20 times as irritating as that of a filter cigaret! Thus, regular use of marijuana worsens your asthma and may even cause COPD or emphysema. Finally, there have also been reports of allergic sensitivity to marijuana itself.

CAN STOVES AND FIREPLACES BE A PROBLEM?

Yes. The use of wood burning stoves (especially without catalytic converters) and old gas stoves, as well as open fireplaces and barbeques, is associated with an increased incidence of asthmatic episodes. The reason is that bothersome levels of irritating sulfur dioxide and particulate substances are emitted from all of these directly into the air you are breathing. Soot itself has been found to markedly worsen asthma.

CAN A SINGLE EXPOSURE TO AN IRRITATING GAS OR SMOKE GIVE ME ASTHMA FOR YEARS?

Yes. Difficulty breathing, coughing, wheezing, and even flu-like symptoms may start within minutes to hours after a single exposure to high concentrations of irritants such as chlorine, smoke, or a "toxic spill." Recently in Richmond, California, there was a spill of oleum, which turns into a cloud of sulfur dioxide and sulfur trioxide when it combines with oxygen in the air. After such a single exposure to a noxious inhalant, you may develop the Reactive Airways Dysfunction Syndrome (RADS), with respiratory symptoms lasting over three months, and subsequently need asthma medications for years, with the possibility of suffering permanent damage to your lungs.

WHAT ABOUT SULFITE PRESERVATIVES?

Various sulfite compounds are commonly used to maintain freshness or appearance in certain foods. Eating a critical amount of the treated food can then precipitate severe and sudden wheezing if you are a susceptible asthmatic. Frequently a trip to the emergency room is necessary. Although small amounts of sulfites are found in foods bought from the grocery, clinically significant amounts are usually only encountered in restaurants. The classical example is the salad bar, where sodium metabisulfite is sprayed on the lettuce to keep it from turning color. Sulfites are also used in beer, wine, and French fries. Guacamole would quickly turn from green to brown without it. The diagnosis can be confirmed with an appropriate challenge by your allergist. Restaurants and supermarkets that use sulfite as an additive should make this fact known to customers. Sulfites in salad bars have been banned in some states. Dried fruits—apricots and apples—contain the highest levels of sulfites and cause serious problems.

WHAT IS THE CHINESE RESTAURANT SYNDROME?

It is ten o'clock at night and you are starving. You go out for Chinese food and during the meal you begin to feel terrible, suffering flushing, palpitations, headache, and sometimes asthma.

This is generally caused by monosodium glutamate (MSG), a protein derivative that functions as a flavor enhancer. It is commonly used in Chinese cooking, but may be found in many other restaurants, including steak houses. The degree to which the syndrome develops is related to the amount of MSG eaten, and the consequences are usually much worse when you are really hungry. Don't be embarrassed—always ask "Please, no MSG."

CAN I DRINK ALCOHOL?

Yes, but in moderation. Whereas the combination of alcohol and antihistamines can act as a dangerous sedative, there is no such harmful interaction between alcohol and bronchodilator medications such as theophylline and metered dose inhalers. Moderate amounts of alcohol do not effect asthma.

You might also be allergic to certain ingredients of alcoholic beverages, such as metabisulfites or the taste-giving congeners in wine. By experimentation, you may be able to identify an alcoholic beverage you can tolerate.

Additionally, drinking alcohol enhances your body's absorption of allergenic food and possibly even inhaled pollen allergens, with obvious consequences. Always, and especially with significant allergies and asthma, moderation in drinking is encouraged. Alcohol may make you careless with severe food allergy.

SEX?

Some asthmatics are greatly disturbed by the wheezing that frequently accompanies lovemaking. Actually, this is just another form of exercise-induced wheezing and may be nothing more than an exacerbation of previously ignored mild asthma. Proper medication can usually control your wheezing, and a spray of bronchodilator before sex may be all that is necessary.

Not to be sensational, but we feel bound to mention here that recent studies show that some women can experience serious allergic reactions to semen, including severe itching and hives, wheezing, and even anaphylactic shock. Latex (rubber) allergy may also cause occasional allergic reactions to condoms.

Is Scuba Diving Compatible with Asthma?

For most people with moderate to severe asthma, the answer is no. This has become an important question in the United States since about 300,000 new divers are certified annually by the PADI (Professional Association of Diving Instructors) organization alone. Until now, asthma has been considered an absolute barrier to scuba diving. The concern is to avoid increasing the risk and incidence of arterial gas embolism (AGE). During scuba (self-contained underwater breathing apparatus) diving, the diver breathes compressed, pressurized air at depths. If you fill a balloon with air from a scuba tank at just 33 feet under water, it will *double* in size when brought to the surface. Thus, upon ascent the air in the scuba diver's bronchial tubes and in the alveoli similarly expands and needs to escape.

All scuba divers must continually breathe upon ascent. If your bronchial tubes are obstructed by the inflammation of asthma, the expanding air has nowhere to escape. It can rupture your bronchioles and alveoli, enter your arterial blood vessels, and be pumped by your heart to your brain and other vital organs. This air in your bloodstream can thus cause severe, life-threatening injuries, and even death.

If you have asthma and wish to scuba dive, consultation and evaluation by an asthma specialist is mandatory. Your allergist or pulmonologist may okay diving if your asthma is completely controlled and your pulmonary functions are normal. The advent of inhaled steroids and Tilade has changed the classic view that no asthmatic can dive, and in fact new clinical studies need to be done to fully confirm this. For the individual asthmatic, however, many factors need to be considered. These include the history of your asthma and its severity, your medication needs, your current trigger factors, your response to breathing cold air, and the location and time of year when you will be diving.

Breathing air from a scuba tank may itself actually trigger asthma. It is known that breathing air that is cold and dry compared to the inside of the bronchial tubes can cause attacks, and since the compressed air in a scuba tank is dry and its temperature is that of the water at the dive site (usually less than your

98 degree body temperature), asthma attacks are readily produced. The decision to scuba dive must be highly individualized and general advice cannot be given.

Free diving is quite unlike scuba diving in its risk to asthmatics. The free diver inhales air at the water's surface that is at atmospheric pressure, and then dives, slightly compressing the air in the lungs. Upon ascent the remaining air can expand only to its original volume, which is obivously not a problem. Asthma patients can therefore enjoy snorkeling, then take in a deep breath, dive down a little, and enjoy the coral and fish.

SHOULD I GET PREGNANT?

Most women with asthma go through pregnancy and delivery without complications, but severe asthmatics risk compromising the health of the fetus. Moreover, complex hormonal changes that occur during pregnancy can also make your asthma better or worse. One-third of pregnant asthmatics will get worse during their pregnancy, one-third will remain the same, and one-third may actually improve. You may need to modify your asthma medications during this period, with close supervision from your physicians.

We have found that asthma does not complicate delivery and many of our most severe (even steroid-dependent) patients have experienced the joy of giving birth to a healthy baby without asthmatic complications and difficulties.

CAN I TAKE ASTHMA MEDICATIONS IF I AM PREGNANT?

You should continue taking your medications, but *only* under your physician's direction. Your physician might prescribe medications such as terbutaline, metaproterenol, albuterol, cromolyn, and inhaled steroids—all of which have been safely used during pregnancy. The preferred inhaled steroid is beclomethasone (Beclovent, Vanceril). If your symptoms are severe, appropriate doses of prednisone may be required. Asthma and allergy-related drugs that should be avoided during pregnancy include adrenalin, the antihistamines brompheniramine, hydroxyzine, and promethazine (many brands), cough preparations containing iodine, and the various tetracyclines. The safety of some newer medications has not been established. Obviously, you should not take more medications than are necessary to control your asthma. The Food and Drug Administration (FDA) has established a safety rating system for the use of drugs in pregnancy. You as an asthmatic should not rely on this rating, but should check with your physician regarding each individual drug you consider taking. Allergic asthmatics often require antihistamines, and chlorpheniramine and pyribenzamine (PBZ) are considered the safest to use.

SHOULD I STOP MY ASTHMA MEDICATIONS IF I AM PREGNANT?

No. This can be dangerous for both you, the mother, and your fetus. If you cannot breathe, the baby cannot breathe because it too will not get adequate oxygen. Untreated asthma can result in low birthweight babies and prematurity.

IS ASTHMA CONTAGIOUS?

Asthma itself is not contagious. Your closest friends are safe and cannot catch your asthma. If your asthma is accompanied by an infection such as influenza, however, you can spread the infection just as anyone might. By the way, since the cold virus is often spread by hand-to-mouth contact, you can protect yourself and others by washing your hands frequently and by using disposable antiseptic tissue.

WHAT IS THE BEST MEDICINE FOR ASTHMA?

The best medicines for your asthma are the ones that give you relief with the fewest side effects. Personal preference is very important. We recommend a stepwise approach in which you first use bronchodilators, which relax your bronchial muscles and open up your airways, and then add the crucially important anti-inflammatory medications.

Treatment depends upon the severity of your asthma. Consensus guidelines for the drug therapy of asthma have been developed by the National Institutes of Health (*see* box on opposite page).

**NIH CONSENSUS GUIDELINES
FOR THE DRUG THERAPY OF ASTHMA**

- *Mild, chronic asthma:* A beta-2 agonist is necessary.
- *Persistent, mild wheezing.* This includes brief intermittent episodes of wheezing and coughing, as well as infrequent wheezing at night: Use anti-inflammatory cromolyn or nedocromil regularly, plus beta-2 agonists, if necessary.
- *Chronic, moderate asthma.* This interferes with lifestyle, requires occasional emergency care, is accompanied by more frequent nocturnal wheezing. Use regular inhaled steroids and/or cromolyn/nedocromil, as well as beta adrenergics as necessary. Consider theophylline. Occasional prednisone may be necessary.
- *Chronic, severe, continuous wheezing.* This limits activities, includes frequent nocturnal asthma, and requires occasional hospitalizations and emergency care. Treatment includes the above medications, and requires high doses of inhaled steroids. Alternate-day prednisone may be necessary.

If your wheezing episodes are mild and infrequent, then inhalation of a bronchodilator delivered by metered dose inhaler is ideal. These inhalers contain a newly developed and expanding group of drugs called beta-2's, such as albuterol (Ventolin, Proventil), metaproterenol (Alupent), terbutaline (Brethaire), bitolterol (Tornalate), and pirbuterol (Maxair). They work fairly rapidly and are generally well tolerated, though some users have experienced such side effects as irritability, tremor, and heart palpitations. The technique of inhalation is critical and your doctor can show you which method is best for you. Devices called "spacers" can dramatically improve delivery and effectiveness.

More useful for ongoing or more severe asthma symptoms is a combination of drugs. For sustained relief from having to use your beta-2 bronchodilator inhaler, it is essential that you also take a medicine to decrease lung inflammation. You need an anti-inflammatory inhaler to deliver either a steroid, or Intal or Tilade. You may additionally need a long-acting bronchodilator

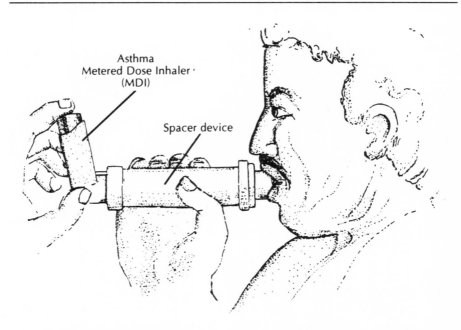

Asthma
Metered Dose Inhaler ·
(MDI)

Spacer device

Spacer device for asthma inhalers traps large, irritating particles while enhancing delivery of medicine to the bronchial tubes.

such as theophylline (Theo-Dur, etc., as sustained-released tablets) in addition to your beta-2 inhaler. If you are clear between episodes of asthma and the beta-2 inhaler alone does not give you enough relief, then you may benefit from a rapidly absorbed but shorter acting theophylline, such as an aminophylline tablet or Elixophyllin liquid. An advantage of theophylline is that it can provide long-term treatment and is easy to take. Disadvantages include the not infrequent complaints of irritability and insomnia, stomach upset, and headaches. Of recent concern is the possibility of difficulty with attention and learning in school children. Because the therapeutic dose is often close to the dangerously toxic dose, individualized dosing is necessary. Viral infections, drugs such as erythromycin, Dilantin, and Tagamet, and liver disease can push the blood levels to the toxic range. Your physician may check your theophylline blood level periodically. Smoking cigarets tends to decrease theophylline blood levels.

Some children benefit from the beta-2 drugs by mouth; metaproterenol (Alupent) and albuterol (Ventolin, Proventil) are frequently used. Though effective and practical, most adults experience a greater number of side effects when beta-2 are drugs taken orally rather than inhaled.

WHAT ARE BETA AGONISTS?

These are adrenalin-like drugs that dilate your bronchial tubes and have minimal cardiac side effects. The most commonly used are albuterol (Proventil, Ventolin), metaproterenol (Alupent), terbutaline (Brethaire), bitolterol (Tornalate), pirbuterol (Maxair); onset of action is rapid. The promising new salmeterol (Serevent) and formoterol provide long-lasting relief. These medications are very safe and helpful, but overuse may lead to dependence and lessened effectiveness.

A "spacer"—Aerochamber or InspirEase—is sometimes necessary for more effective delivery of these metered-dose inhaler medications. Such spacers have proved important for the young, the elderly, and for those with severe asthma. Home nebulizers for use with beta-2 agonist medications have also been very helpful for young children and many adults, although proper use of a metered dose inhaler in conjunction with the spacer is usually just as effective and more reasonably managed.

Excessive use of your beta-2 agonist inhaler (more than four to six times a day) means that your asthma is poorly controlled and you should contact your physician immediately. Such excessive use allows the inflammation to continue and worsen and has been associated with increased deaths from asthma—again, because the asthma is so severe and further emergency medications do not provide timely relief.

Oral, long-acting beta-2 agonists (Proventil, 4 milligram Repetabs, Volmax, 4 and 8 milligrams) can be very helpful for your asthma when it flares at 3 AM. Such nocturnal asthma can be dangerous and life-threatening.

Isuprel and the over-the-counter medicines Primatene mist and Bronkaid will give you the fastest relief from asthma. Although Olympic athletes can be seen endorsing over-the-counter inhalers, cardiac side effects are very common and the improvement of bronchial relaxation they provide lasts only a very short time, requiring frequently repeated doses while the inflammation continues. Your asthma should be controlled well enough so that you will not seek out these adrenalin inhalers.

WHAT ABOUT THE DRUG THAT PREVENTS WHEEZING?

Intal (cromolyn sodium) and the new Tilade (nedocromil) work in any age group by preventing the spasm that produces wheezing and by decreasing the inflammation of the bronchial tubes. They are especially useful for moderately asthmatic patients and in the prevention of exercise-induced wheezing. Nedocromil is also helpful in dealing with the asthma caused by irritants and pollutants, for post-seasonal pollen asthma, and for reducing the dosage of inhaled steroids in more severe asthmatics. Their great advantage is the absence of any behavioral, cardiac, or gastrointestinal side effects. Remember, they are not bronchodilators and will not relieve an acute episode. In order to be effective Intal or Tilade must be used regularly. Intal is available as a metered dose inhaler, an inhaled powder-capsule with a spinhaler, and a solution for a home nebulizer; Tilade as a metered dose inhaler. Though Intal and Tilade are very helpful for those with moderate asthma, inhaled steroids are the stronger anti-inflammatory drugs needed by those with severe asthma.

ARE STEROIDS DANGEROUS?

Corticosteroids such as prednisone and Medrol are essential in treating severe asthma and other allergic conditions such as nasal allergy, hives, eczema, and sinusitis. Without these medications there would be far more disability and death from asthma. Unfortunately, many of the side effects caused by corticosteroids can be dangerous (*see* box on opposite page). Most of these side effects are related to dosage and can be avoided by careful control of the usage of these medications. Inhaled corticosteroid preparations such as beclomethasone (Vanceril, Beconase, Vancenase, Beclovent), triamcinolone (Azmacort), flunisolide (Aerobid, Nasalide) are not significantly absorbed into the body's blood-

---

SIDE EFFECTS OF ORAL OR INJECTED CORTICOSTEROIDS

- Increased appetite and weight gain
- Puffiness of the face
- Aggravation of underlying diabetes or rarely a diabetic-type condition
- Osteoporosis (thinning of the bones)
- Linear growth retardation and delayed puberty in children
- Cataracts
- Emotional changes
- Skin changes such as easy bruising and acne
- Decreased resistance to infection
- Loss of blood flow to the large bone in the hip requiring later hip replacement
- Gastrointestinal problems such as heartburn, or rarely ulceration
- High blood pressure
- Low potassium, which can cause muscle cramps

---

stream when used as directed in the usual dosage range. Therefore they do not cause the severe side effects that can occur with either oral or injected corticosteroids. With respect to inhaled steroids for asthma, most clinical investigators feel that up to 16 sprays (12 for children) of Vanceril or Azmacort per day should be safe for long-term use.

Oral or injected corticosteroids are used when your asthma does not respond to other medications or could potentially be life-threatening. Inhaled corticosteroids may not work well when your symptoms are severe and are more useful for the prevention of chronic asthma or allergy symptoms. The lowest possible dose and the shortest treatment course of corticosteroids should be used to control your asthma and thereby diminish the likelihood of side effects. If prolonged steroid treatment with prednisone is necessary, every effort should be made to achieve an alternate-day dosing schedule.

It is important also to be aware that short doses of oral systemic steroids—even for three to four days—can result in emotional lability. Some asthmatics report that they feel a little "crazy" when they take oral systemic steroids for even these short periods. There is often difficulty with sleeping, as well as agitation or depression. It is essential that patients take corticosteroids only when recommended by their physician and then follow instructions carefully. Notify your physician if you feel you are having symptoms of any of these side effects.

WILL THE STEROIDS I TAKE FOR ASTHMA AND ALLERGY GIVE ME GREAT MUSCLES?

No. The term "steroid" refers to a large group of hormones secreted internally in the body by the adrenal glands and the gonads—the testes and the ovaries. Steroids as a class of substances also include the related drug compounds manufactured and used for therapy.

The steroids necessary for your asthma therapy are in an entirely different category. Prednisone does *not* give you the muscle strength and endurance that come from the "anabolic" steroids used to artificially build muscles for sports competition—in fact, they produce just the opposite effects, weakness and wasting. Anabolic steroids are related to the male hormone androgen (testosterone); they can have dangerous cardiovascular side effects and are also implicated in some cancers. On the other hand, prednisone is an anti-inflammatory and reduces swelling from allergy and infection.

CAN THERE BE COMPLICATIONS WITH CHICKENPOX WHEN I AM TAKING STEROIDS?

Possibly. In children chickenpox is an exceedingly uncomfortable, but a self-limited and relatively benign disease without complications. In patients whose immune systems have been suppressed by cancer and anticancer drugs, by AIDS, by congenital immunodeficiency, and perhaps by long-term, high-dose oral or injected steroids, chickenpox may be a serious and perhaps life-threatening illness since the virus will be able to spread unhindered throughout the body.

There may be a small, theoretical risk associated with the use of short-term systemic steroids, and an even smaller one with inhaled steroids. The incubation period for chickenpox is approximately three weeks. If you or your child have asthma that either has, or may, require systemic or inhaled steroids, let your doctor know immediately. If you are taking oral steroids, you can, within two days after exposure, still receive gamma globulin-containing antibodies to the chickenpox virus and prevent the incubation. If you do not receive gamma immune globulin, an antiviral drug acyclovir, can be used to lessen your chickenpox symptoms.

Remember to keep your child away from his or her trigger factors. Get the cat out, increase the your or your child's dose of Intal or Tilade, and perhaps of the beta agonist, albuterol. Do not deviate from your asthma control plan. You may mistakenly substitute a life-threatening, severe asthma episode for a theoretical risk of steroid or other side effects.

WHY DON'T MY INHALED STEROIDS WORK?

Inhaled steroids reduce lung inflammation over a period of days. They do not immediately open up your airways. You must take them regularly, and if you are prescribed more than eight inhalations total per day, then you should take the inhaled steroid in three or four divided doses. The timing between these doses is not important—you can wait until you get home from school or work. These inhaled steroids are safe—very little is absorbed and what is absorbed is rapidly broken down in your liver. The most commonly observed side effect with inhaled steroids is hoarseness; a bothersome yeast infection can also occur. Both of these side effects can be minimized by appropriate use of a spacer with the metered-dose inhaler steroid. It is also important to rinse your mouth with water after using your inhaled steroid. While there is certainly some significant absorption of steroid at high doses—more than 16 inhalations for adults and 12 for children—the benefit in severe asthma is striking when compared to the risks of undertreatment. Remember, your inhaled steroids save you from the side effects of higher doses of

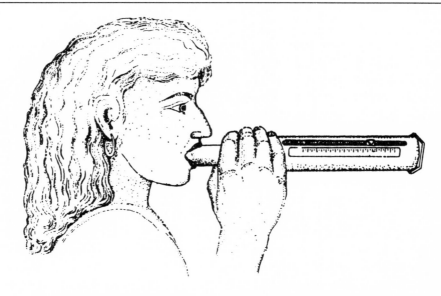

Monitoring asthma control using a personal peak flow meter.

prednisone. Be sure to take your inhaled steroid on a regular schedule; they will not work in an emergency!

Do I Need a Peak Flow Meter?

Yes. A peak flow meter is essential to monitor the course of your asthma if you require beta agonist bronchodilator medications on a regular basis. By establishing your personal best value, you and your allergist can establish an asthma control plan. Even if you are observant, your asthma condition may be more severe than you realize. Asthmatics often become used to breathing with a very low lung function and the peak flow meter can identify the need for timely medications. This is the best way to document your lung function on a day to day basis at home so that your physician can appropriately adjust your medications.

It is also important to avoid excessive use of such bronchodilator medications as albuterol. You and your physician should establish your personal best expiratory flow rate, and jointly agree your bronchodilator inhaler should not be necessary when your rate is above 85% of that personal best value even

PREDICTED AVERAGE PEAK FLOW FOR NORMAL MALE AND FEMALE CHILDREN		
Age	Height	Peak flow
5	43"	145
7	47–48"	200–220
12	59–60"	350–387
15	64–66"	420–460

PREDICTED AVERAGE PEAK FLOW FOR NORMAL MALES AND FEMALES								
Males					Females			
	Height					·Height		
Age	60"	65"	70"	75"	Age	55"	65"	70"	75"
20	554	602	649	693	20	390	460	496	529
30	532	577	622	664	30	380	448	483	516
40	509	552	596	636	40	370	436	470	502
50	486	527	569	607	50	360	424	457	488

if you are feeling some degree of mild asthma. Excessive, unnecessary use of your bronchodilator inhaler may result in actual increased need for more bronchodilator dosages. Your lungs literally get used to needing the inhaler and require more frequent treatment. Even with exercise-induced asthma, it is not always necessary to use your bronchodilator. Appropriate "warming up" and "warming down" maneuvers can be helpful.

HOW CAN I DETERMINE MY PERSONAL BEST PEAK FLOW VALUE?

The range of "normal" peak flows is broad and dependent upon your age and height. The following values are given only so you know "you are in the right ballpark." For a seven-year-old who is 47 inches tall, a peak flow of 100 always needs attention, but the child's normal no-asthma value may be about 180–220.

We would define your personal best as the peak flow value obtained when you and your physician determine that your asthma is under practical and reasonable good control. On high-dose steroids some patients may be able to achieve a temporary high peak-flow value, but this value is not meaningful in monitoring your day-to-day medications. Peak-flow measurements are effort dependent, so try two or three times for each determination. If the three peak flow readings are not close to each other, the low value may represent poor effort. A short and quick breath produces the best peak flow. Fill your lungs until they feel they are going to burst and then blow rapidly into the peak flow meter. Practice is essential. A long and slow breath won't even move the peak flow meter.

It is important to be aware that the actual peak flow readings may vary significantly among peak flow meters, so use the same peak flow meter for each reading. Also, be aware that your own peak flow meter reading may vary from the one you used in your physician's office.

WHAT IS AN ASTHMA CONTROL PLAN?

An asthma control plan is necessary for control of moderate to severe asthma and it is best based on peak flow monitoring (*see* box on opposite page).

Low oxygen levels in the blood associated with asthma results in an increased heart rate and increased number of breaths per minute (respiratory rate). The upper limit of normal for heart rate is 140 for children and 120 for adults; and the upper limit of normal for the respiratory rate is 30 breaths per minute.

WHAT SHOULD I EXPECT IN THE EMERGENCY ROOM?

First and most importantly, the Emergency Room physician will assess your current condition, including:

- Your medical history, including the names and dosages of all medications, will be taken (keep a list in your wallet or purse at all times; or bring your medications with you).

ASTHMA CONTROL PLAN

Essential elements:
- Recognition of trigger factors, allergens, infections, pollutants
- Environmental control measures for dust, molds, pets
- Peak flows daily or as necessary for exacerbations
- A written list of medications, based on percentage of your personal best peak flow values
- Tells you when to call your physician or when to go to the Emergency Room

The specifics are individualized by your physician; however, there are certain basic guidelines for emergency care:

- Peak flow less than 50% of your established personal best
- Poor color
- Listlessness
- Paradoxical stomach movement (i.e., the stomach goes out, instead of in, when breathing out)
- Severe shortness of breath with rapid breathing
- Poor or little response to your inhaled beta agonist

- A physical examination, including listening to your chest and measuring your blood pressure and heart rate, will be carried out
- Measurement of your lung function by a pulmonary function test
- Measurement of your blood oxygen, and carbon dioxide if necessary
- Chest X-ray when necessary
- Laboratory studies on your blood: red and white counts, serum potassium, theophylline

After assessment, your treatment may include:

- Oxygen
- Nebulized beta agonist: continuous if severe
- Injected beta agonist: terbutaline or adrenalin
- Injected corticosteroids

At this point, it is hoped you will be sufficiently improved to be able to go home. Your peak flow should approach 70% of your personal best. Remember to keep in close contact with the physician monitoring your asthma. Even though you have been treated with injectable steroids, remember to continue your inhaled steroids.

WHICH DRUGS MUST I AVOID IF I HAVE ASTHMA?

Certain drugs can trigger an attack in asthmatic patients. Such episodes may have a sudden onset with long duration and great severity. Beta-blockers (*not* beta-agonists) are a class of drugs commonly used to treat heart conditions and high blood pressure, as well as migraine headaches, hyperthyroid disorders, and, topically, glaucoma. Your asthma may flare up seriously if you use them, so be alert to the possibility. If you have hay fever, these drugs may precipitate latent asthma, especially during a heavy pollen season. Among many beta-blockers, some examples are: propanolol (Inderal), metoprolol (Lopressor), nadolol (Corgard), atenolol (Tenormin), and the eyedrops timolol (Timoptic) and betaxolol (Betoptic).

Aspirin should probably also be avoided if you suffer chronic asthma. Up to 10% of adults and children with asthma become worse when they take aspirin. This adverse reaction to aspirin can occur at any age, even if you were able to tolerate it previously. Interestingly, this reaction appears after 20 to 30 minutes. Asthmatics particularly at risk for aspirin-sensitivity are a subgroup with a history of chronic sinusitis and perhaps nasal polyps. Although their respiratory symptoms may be severe, they usually do not have typical allergic sensitivities to pollens, molds, and other allergens. Medications chemically related to aspirin should also be avoided if you are sensitive to aspirin. These include many of the anti-inflammatory drugs used for arthritis, musculoskeletal pain, and backache. The list is very long and includes ibuprofen (Advil, Nuprin, Motrin, Relafen), naproxen (Naprosyn, Anaprox), piroxicam (Feldene), and ketorolac (Toradol). Physicians and pharmacists refer to this group of anti-inflammatory drugs as NSAIDs—nonsteroidal anti-inflammatory drugs. Be sure to check with your physician if you have aspirin sensitivity before taking any medications.

MAY I PLAY SPORTS?

Would you like to win an Olympic medal? For the first time in the 1984 Summer Olympics in Los Angeles, 66 US competitors had asthma (10% of the US Olympians). Forty-one won medals: 15 gold, 21 silver, and five bronze. The swimmers excelled. The days of asthmatics being restricted from participation in sports activities are gone. With newer medicines and treatments for asthma, you stand an equal chance to come out a winner. The key to winning is control of your asthma by doing everything your physician tells you to do, and taking the prescribed medicines before competing.

Exercise should be an essential part of the overall care of your asthma. If you can tolerate it, aerobic exercise is ideal. Aerobic exercise includes running, swimming, and energetic dancing. These exercises improve the ability of muscles to use oxygen efficiently, thus increasing your endurance. Many asthmatics tolerate swimming best. Exercise-induced bronchospasm and wheezing are triggered by breathing air that is relatively cold and dry compared to the air in the bronchial tubes. But the swimmer breathes air that is well humidified and is at the temperature of the warm water. With less than optimal control you may choose a less strenuous activity such as bowling, golf, and light weight training. *See* box on next page for tips for controlling your exercise-induced wheezing.

WHAT ABOUT BACKPACKING?

Backpacking may result in your exposure to excessive quantities of pollens at certain times of the year. If you are allergic to grass, don't backpack on a valley floor in April, May, and June. However, immunotherapy with allergy shots can help alleviate the problem, and you should consider this possibly preventive course. If the exertion of backpacking itself triggers wheezing, then an appropriate bronchodilator, cromolyn, or nedocromil (Tilade) should be used beforehand. You should not avoid this

> **TIPS FOR CONTROLLING YOUR EXERCISE-INDUCED WHEEZING**
> - Keep your asthma generally under good control
> - Use Intal or Tilade before exercise
> - Use your beta agonist as necessary either before, during, or after exercise
> - Try a short warm-up period, rest, and then exercise
> - Take a short break and breathe through your nose
> - Try a slow warm-down after vigorous exercise
> - Use inhaled steroids or Tilade to prevent the wheezing that occurs hours after your exercise is completed

excellent physical outdoor activity; however, severe asthmatics should *not* be isolated from emergency medical services. Take a supply of prednisone with you, if you have in the past ever needed steroid medications to control your asthma.

SHOULD I GO TO ASTHMA CAMP?

There are several camps that provide educational and recreational programs for asthma patients. And, there are many children who will need the special medical support provided only at such a camp. These programs teach the children topics about asthma, including its causes, prevention, and treatments. The participant is encouraged to enjoy the various recreational activities that also help to build self-esteem and confidence. The camp additionally provides a welcome break for the tired parent caregiver and a chance to regroup and get a fresh start. Although there are obvious advantages to such a camp, not all are willing to participate because being at a special camp for asthmatics may reinforce the disheartening concept that having asthma places you in a category of "not normal" people. You may also find, if your child's asthma is mild, that such a camp is really not necessary.

Whether your child should go to an asthma camp must be an individual decision, but you should ask your physician for advice when considering this matter.

FACTORS THAT PREDISPOSE YOU TO LIFE-THREATENING ASTHMA

- Severe nocturnal asthma: flareups at 3 or 4 AM
- Previous life-threatening flareups of asthma with Emergency Room visits and/or hospitalizations
- Frequent need for systemic steroids such as prednisone
- Emotional and psychological problems, especially when asthma provides the patient with more attention
- Inner city socioeconomic disadvantage
- Statistically higher incidence in a subpopulation, e.g., Afro-Americans
- Advancing age: over 55 years
- Aspirin and sulfite sensitivity
- Underestimating the severity of your asthma and remaining unaware of the dangers—denial and complacency

CAN I DIE FROM ASTHMA?

Yes. Asthma can be fatal (*see* box) and the number of deaths from asthma is increasing worldwide. In a US city with a population of 500,000, from five to ten asthmatics may be expected to succumb from their disease each year. This information is not reported to frighten you, but only to reinforce the notion that the proper use of improved medications with close medical supervision is necessary if we are to keep mortality an uncommon occurrence. Early and aggressive treatment minimizes the risk of fatal complications. You may need the intensive care available in a hospital. In spite of the potential mortality, asthmatics do have a normal life expectancy.

SHOULD I MOVE?

Moving to a different city and environment may be of benefit if there will be less air pollution. Moving to avoid heavy pollen areas is not advisable. After a few seasons you are likely to develop new pollen allergies. Mold allergy asthmatics often benefit from relocating to a drier climate. Many have less difficulty with wheezing when they move to an area with a more moderate climate.

Some allergens are unique and more prevalent in certain regions. With modern asthma control plans, you should be able to live comfortably in most areas you might choose.

CAN ASTHMA BE CURED?

Asthma can be controlled, but bronchial tubes often remain irritable even after symptoms subside. Therefore, the disease may persist and may always require attention. When the cat is removed, the wheezing stops—but the asthma remains.

4

Skin Allergy

4 SKIN ALLERGY

KNOWN CAUSES OF URTICARIA

- Drugs (*see* bottom of page)
- Insect stings
- Foods
- Food additives
- Infections
- Parasites
- Colds
- Exercise
- Lupus erythematosus
- Cancer (rarely)
- Physical urticaria—cold, pressure/friction, contact with water, body heat, photosensitivity, vibration

---

WHAT ARE HIVES?

"Hives" is the common word for the dermatological condition formally known as *urticaria*, which is characterized by itchy "bumps" in the skin that vary from pinhead size to welts several inches across. The hive (or *wheal*) is raised and pale and is usually surrounded by an area of redness and warmth (*erythema*).

Normal skin is peppered with mast cells, which contain histamine. The allergic reaction releases histamine into your skin, irritating nerve endings, and thus causing itching. Histamine also causes tiny blood vessels in your skin to dilate and ooze clear serum. The serum swells and raises your skin, resulting in the wheal, and your dilated blood vessels produce the erythema and warmth of the hive.

WHAT CAUSES HIVES?

Urticaria has many causes (*see* box). Searching for the cause of urticaria is frustrating detective work for both the patient and the allergist. Unfortunately, in most cases, the cause may never be found. Stress is often an important factor.

WHAT MEDICATIONS CAUSE HIVES?

The list is extensive, including most, if not all, medications. The prime offenders are:

- Penicillin
- Sulfa antibiotics and chemically related diuretics

- Nonsteroidal anti-inflammatory drugs (NSAIDs) such as aspirin and ibuprofen
- Codeine
- Barbiturates (phenobarbital)

Your hives can occur immediately upon taking the medicine you are allergic to, or can start up to six weeks after the medication has been stopped. Additionally, you can develop hives after taking your medication without problems for years.

Is Diet Important in Hives?

Food allergy is one of the most frequent causes of acute hives. Many foods are known to cause urticaria, although each patient is usually allergic to only one or two such foods. The list includes fish or shellfish, nuts, peanuts, and eggs. Prepared foods may contain these dangerously "hidden" ingredients. Dairy products may also be responsible. If you have hives, you should always avoid tomatoes and strawberries as well as alcoholic beverages since these can accentuate your hives even if they are not the prime cause.

Food additives are sometimes suspect. In many cases, coal-tar derived compounds, such as yellow dye No. 5 (tartrazine yellow) might be responsible. This additive is ubiquitous in our diet, especially in orange-flavored foods. It is used to make foods appear to be rich in eggs and also to color some butter and margarine. Even fresh oranges have been injected with tartrazine to improve their color! Some preservatives such as benzoates (BHT and BHA) can cause urticaria. Trace amounts of antibiotics in food may also be responsible for hives. This has occurred when allergics sensitive to penicillin drank milk from penicillin-treated cows.

Are Hives Seasonal?

Yes, patients who are allergic to pollens have more difficulty with hives during the pollen season. Additionally, contact with grass may result in hives. Infrequently, hives may be caused by allergic sensitivity to inhalants such as dust mites. Bringing pets into your house may cause urticaria flareups in the winter.

ARE HIVES CAUSED BY NERVES?

Hives are frequently blamed on nerves. As in many illnesses, it is easy to say it is caused by "nerves" when the real physical cause is unknown or difficult to unmask. Not all "nervous" people have hives, but many allergics tell us that their hives are worse when they are nervous and under stress. Indeed, emotional upset or trauma can result in a flareups of hives, but the development of urticaria does not necessarily mean you need counseling. It is actually a group of chemical substances in the nerve endings—the neuropeptides—that cause your hives, as well as hay fever, asthma, and ulcers; your body releases these neuropeptides in response to your various emotional stimuli.

CAN THE SUN CAUSE HIVES?

Yes. Physical factors such as the energy of sunlight can cause urticaria. Avoidance of sunlight and the use of sunscreens such as Shade and UVA Guard can prevent hives. A new product that physically blocks the rays is very effective—titanium dioxide. There is no cure for sun-caused hives, beyond the avoidance of sunlight exposure to your skin.

Conversely, exposure to cold temperatures may also result in urticaria, a condition that may be inherited. The medication Periactin is considered the best prevention for cold urticaria. Allergics with cold-induced hives should take care to determine their tolerance to cold water. Those who are very sensitive may develop frank life-threatening anaphylaxis if they jump into a cold lake or pool.

CAN SUN BLOCKERS CAUSE ALLERGY?

Yes. Allergy to the most common sunscreen, PABA (para-aminobenzoic acid), and to the related compound padimate O, are quite common. Since the energy of sunlight causes these compounds to combine with skin proteins, the response these produce is called photoallergic. The PABA–protein complex produced sensitizes the skin and a reaction similar to that occurring with poison oak results. But only when PABA is placed on the skin of a person sensitive to it does exposure to the sun set off the reaction.

Photoallergic reactions to oxybenzone, a replacement for PABA, are now unfortunately becoming common. A newer agent, avobenzone, can also block ultraviolet A (UVA) light. Already allergic reactions to it have been reported.

Sunburn, premature aging of the skin, skin cancer, and some sun-sensitizing reactions are caused mainly by exposure to that portion of solar radiation known as ultraviolet B (UVB). Most sun-related drug reactions (photosensitizing) are caused by exposure to the longer wavelength UVA rays. These UVA rays tan the skin; but UVA also causes sunburn and skin damage. Thus, UVA exposure can set off a disconcerting red, raised rash of varying severity over the exposed areas of the skin—polymorphous skin eruptions.

Avobenzone and oxybenzone help to block both UVA and UVB radiation. A sunscreen that blocks UVB only—octyl-methoxycinnamate—may cause fewer allergic reactions.

If you develop a reaction to a sunscreen, write down the ingredients of the offending product. Many prescriptions contain more than one sunscreen. Then choose a new brand containing different sunscreens, which may be difficult if you want UVA protection. Micropulverized titanium dioxide physically blocks all sun rays, and since it does not combine with your skin proteins, should not cause photoallergic reactions. Titanium dioxide preparations may also contain the allergenic sunscreens, so read the list of ingredients carefully.

CAN I JOG AND TAKE A SAUNA WITH HIVES?

Physical activity and stress precipitate attacks of hives; indeed, any exercise may exacerbate your urticaria. Sauna baths and hot tubs may prove intolerable. One type, known as cholinergic urticaria, is specifically caused by an increase in your body heat and exercise. The tiny hives it produces are treated with Atarax (hydroxyzine).

Exercise anaphylaxis occurs when you engage in such aerobic exercise as jogging. Its symptoms can include trouble breathing and low blood pressure, as well as hives. Food allergy may be an additional aggravating factor. A nonsedating antihistamine (Seldane, Hismanal, Claritin) may be helpful, and you should keep an emergency adrenalin kit available if you are susceptible.

ARE HIVES DANGEROUS?

Your hives are not dangerous in themselves, but hives may be a warning of a more serious generalized anaphylactic reaction. Urticaria is sometimes associated with a swelling of your lips, tongue, and throat, a condition known as *angioedema*. Angioedema of your larynx (voice box) constitutes a medical emergency requiring adrenalin. Sometimes a tracheostomy is necessary to open a passage for air in the windpipe. If you suffer from cold urticaria, simply jumping into cold water or drinking a cold liquid may cause an allergic reaction whose symptoms include hives.

Hereditary angioedema is a rare and, when untreated, potentially fatal disease involving swelling of the face, larynx, intestines, and extremities. The swelling does not itch, but is very painful. Fortunately, blood tests can easily provide the diagnosis, and the condition can then be controlled by very small doses of synthetic hormones related to the male hormone, *testosterone*. Adrenalin usually does not help. Acute attacks can be treated by replacing your deficient serum proteins with infusions of fresh frozen plasma, whole blood transfusions, and most appropriately, with a concentrate of the actual missing enzyme inhibitor (not yet available in the United States). A tracheostomy is sometimes necessary.

CAN A SKIN RASH CAUSE DEATH?

Yes. Mastocytosis is a rare condition in which an exaggerated number of mast cells that contain histamine are stored deep in the body organs. When an allergic mastocytotis rash is present, many of the mast cells can be found in the skin lesions. The rash is rough and reddish brown, and symptoms include will itchy flushing, headaches, nasal symptoms, stomach acidity, and psychological problems. Severe anaphylactic shock and death can follow. A biopsy is diagnostic.

Mastocytosis usually starts in childhood and may spontaneously subside; when it first appears in adults, it is more likely to be serious. If you have mastocytosis, you should avoid alcohol and stress. Antihistamines are helpful, and Gastrocrom (cromolyn sodium) may be necessary for your intestinal problems.

ARE THERE SKIN TESTS FOR MY HIVES?

In some cases, limited skin tests can determine that a specific food or inhalant allergen leads to your hives. Skin tests can help diagnose penicillin allergy, but are not useful with other drugs. Skin testing can diagnose allergy to bee stings, a cause of sudden urticaria. An ice cube test is done for cold-induced hives. A thorough medical history by your allergist remains the best diagnostic tool in determining whether you have hives.

WILL MY DOCTOR FIND THE CAUSE OF MY HIVES?

Most likely, no. Be well advised that 90% of the time your physician will not be able to find the cause of your hives if they have been present for six weeks or longer. A routine health check, minimal blood tests, and specific skin tests when indicated by history are recommended. Very specific tests that mimic the conditions causing flareups of hives—a vibration test, sunlight, an ice cube test, and heat—may confirm the cause of your hives. Remember that food challenges should be undertaken very cautiously, and only when there is a doubt regarding certain foods. Do not challenge yourself with a food such as peanuts or shellfish when you are sure that this food causes a severe reaction. If you fall into that 90% of allergics who do not find causes for their hives, don't be frustrated; instead, direct your energies into avoiding exacerbating factors and working out an optimal medications plan with your allergist. Remember, spontaneous remissions from hives do recur, and a large percentage of sufferers can expect their hives to clear up within three to five years.

ATOPIC DERMATITIS

Clinical features:
- Itchiness (pruritus) and dryness of the skin
- Chronic, persistent rash
- Family history of allergy

Characteristic physical distributions of eczema:
- Infancy—face, arms, and knees
- Children—folds of the arms and legs
- Adults—hands, feet, and neck

CAN MEDICATION CURE HIVES?

No. Medications are very helpful, however, in controlling the symptoms of your urticaria. Antihistamines are the drugs of choice; chlorpheniramine (Chlor-Trimeton), diphenhydramine (Benadryl), and hydroxyzine (Atarax) are commonly used. New non-sedating antihistamines include Seldane, Hismanal, and Claritin. Specific recommendations include Periactin for your cold urticaria and Atarax for your cholinergic urticaria.

Another class of antihistamines that decrease stomach acid, but do not treat hay fever includes Tagamet, Zantac, and Pepcid. These can be very helpful when taken together with classical antihistamines. For severe refractory cases, some allergics benefit from doxepin, which in high doses is an antidepressant, but in low doses is an effective antihistamine. Acute, severe attacks may be helped by adrenalin. Your physician may also try oral adrenalin-like drugs. Cortisone may be added for short-term control in severe cases, and sometimes it is necessary to continue prednisone indefinitely with an alternate-day regimen.

WHAT IS ECZEMA?

Eczema is a skin eruption that is itchy, red, and dry. This condition may be acute or chronic.

The chronic type of eczema that is observed in the early years of life is commonly called *atopic dermatitis* (*see* box) and frequently occurs in highly allergic patients. Up to 10% of children and 1% of adults have atopic dermatitis. Approximately one-third of pediatric eczema patients have well-defined allergic causes such as foods and sometimes inhalant allergens (dust mites and grass pollen). These individuals frequently develop respiratory allergies, such as hay fever and asthma as they mature.

The acute forms of eczema include poison oak, skin infections, metal contact sensitivities, detergent irritations, and pityriasis rosea, a severe but transient rash of unknown cause.

Is Eczema Always Allergic?

Not always. Stress can result in a scratch–itch cycle. Eczema also causes a great deal of stress and children especially should be carefully counseled that their eczema can improve. Your eczema can occur in response to exposures to a variety of nonallergic irritating substances such as detergents and industrial chemicals (irritant contact dermatitis). It can also be seen as a reaction to chronic scratching (neurodermatitis) and it generally gets worse when you perspire heavily.

Allergic eczema results from exposure to an allergen that produces a specific immune response, and is categorized as either atopic dermatitis or contact dermatitis. Further discussion of eczema will be limited to atopic dermatitis.

Skin testing to foods is a valuable tool for the diagnosis of the possible allergic triggers of your eczema. The most frequent food causes are peanuts, eggs, milk, wheat, shrimp, soybean, and fish.

Is Eczema Infectious?

No. But skin affected by eczema generally becomes infected very easily. The excessive dryness that is produced by poor skin management—prolonged bathing and inadequate moisturizers—can leave your skin intolerably itchy. The breakage of your skin that results from scratching itchy areas then allows bacteria to enter. Signs of significant skin infection include increased weeping, crusting, and swelling. Once the infection begins, it can spread from a localized area to become a generalized skin infection.

The invading bacteria are usually "staph" *(Staphylococcus)* and occasionally "strep" *(Streptococcus)*. These organisms must be eradicated with systemically administered antibiotics as soon as possible. Erythromycin is most commonly used. If the infection is resistant to erythromycin, however, it may require dicloxacillin or clindamycin. Additionally, some eczema sufferers require long-term preventive antibiotic therapy. A locally applied antibiotic ointment, Bactroban, is very helpful.

Good hygiene and control of your itching are critical in the prevention of serious skin infections.

WHAT PARTS OF THE BODY DOES ECZEMA AFFECT?

All parts of the body can be affected by eczema, but noticeable lesions tend to develop in those areas where the individual is most likely to reach and scratch.

During infancy, the cheeks and the skin behind the ears are affected first. Then, the eczema lesions may "spread" to the forehead and outer surfaces of the arms and legs. The folds of the elbows and knees, the ankles and wrists, and sides of the neck are classic sites for subsequent involvement. Dust mite allergy can cause eczema on exposed skin—don't sit on the carpet!

CAN I BE VACCINATED IF I HAVE ECZEMA OR FOOD ALLERGY?

Smallpox vaccination, when it was used, was never allowed for allergics because of the severe and fatal complications that could and did occur in such individuals. Fortunately, smallpox vaccination is a thing of the past. Other vaccinations such as the childhood immunization shots to pertussis (whooping cough), diphtheria, tetanus, mumps, measles, rubella (German measles), and *Hemophilus b.* (meningitis) are permissible.

Be sure to let your doctor know if you are allergic to eggs. The MMR vaccine (measles, mumps, rubella [German measles]) may contain traces of egg protein. If a child is so allergic to eggs that they cannot be eaten (the skin-test for eggs would be positive), then the child should be skin tested by an allergist with a dilute solution of the vaccine to be used. If the test is positive, a desensitization using multiple small doses of the vaccine may be necessary. Since the vaccine is essentially pure, most egg-sensitive patients will tolerate it. Flu shots should not be given to individuals with egg allergy. Pneumonia and polio vaccines are okay.

DOES ECZEMA CHANGE WITH AGE?

Eczema can begin and resolve spontaneously at any age. In most patients, eczema is apparent by the age of two years. It may be seen, however, as early as the second month of life.

Infantile eczema usually clears spontaneously. Some may continue to be afflicted throughout their childhood years. The sites of involvement change from the face to the arms and legs as the child grows, and childhood eczema often clears by puberty. A child has a 50% chance of outgrowing his eczema by the age of two years or a 75% chance by puberty.

Adult eczema can be present in various patterns, appearing most commonly on the hands, feet, and neck.

IS ECZEMA ASSOCIATED WITH ASTHMA?

There is a strong correlation between asthma and a history of childhood eczema. It has been reported that, based on retrospective studies, one-third of the eczema patients with a family history of allergies will develop asthma.

If your child has eczema, you may be able to prevent later serious allergies such as asthma. You should continue to exclude known food allergens from the child's diet. Nutramigen—not soy milk—is the best substitute for children allergic to cow's milk. Why substitute another potential allergen—soybean—for cow's milk protein? Don't ask for problems by bringing pets into your house, by using feather pillows, or by allowing your child to sleep in a dusty room.

WILL MY ECZEMA GET WORSE IN COLD CLIMATES?

You can expect your eczema to worsen in a colder climate, especially at higher altitudes where the air contains less moisture, making your skin dry and itchy. At low temperatures, you might also be tempted to wear wool clothing, which can further irritate the skin. On the other hand, many eczematics find that their eczema completely clears when they go to tropical areas.

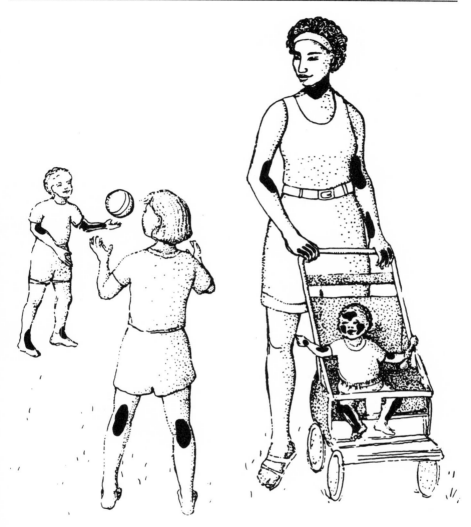

Sites of eczema.

CAN MY DOG BE THE CAUSE OF MY ECZEMA?

Yes! And other pets can cause it, too. You might not observe any obvious association between dog exposure and the worsening of your skin condition. However, if skin tests show that you are sensitive to dog allergen, you may only need to come in contact with dried dog saliva or small amounts of dander left in the living room to cause your eczema flare up. The same rule also applies to other animals such as cats, hamsters, mice, and horses.

CAN ORANGE JUICE MAKE MY ECZEMA WORSE?

Yes. When orange juice contacts eczematous skin, there is usually irritation. Foods one frequently associates with eczema include eggs, peanuts, cow's milk, soybean, wheat, fish, shrimp, chicken, and pork. When properly carried out, trial elimination diets will identify the foods that make the eczema flare up. Skin testing is a definite help.

WHY DO I ITCH SO MUCH WITH MY ECZEMA?

Everybody feels a little itch most of the time. If you think about it, your skin itches in a few places right now; but this is usually ignored. Normal skin becomes more itchy with excessive dryness, especially with the frequent use of soaps in the winter.

If you have eczema, the itch is more intense and your response to stimuli is exaggerated. Dry skin is the most important factor in eczema, and your itchiness and the skin's dryness go hand in hand. Mechanical irritants such as wool and polyesters are major sources of difficulty for eczema patients.

Scratching, which may bring temporary relief, is a normal response to an itch, but does more harm than good. Scratching your dry, scaly skin will lead to infection and result in cracked, weeping lesions and subsequent scarring. This infected skin makes the eczematic's itch become even more intense. Because of the altered state of immunity in eczema patients, skin infections are more common. Trimming fingernails, especially in eczematic children, is advisable.

WHAT SHOULD I WEAR WITH MY ECZEMA?

Ideally, nothing, but the best clothing is of loose-fitting cotton. This is the least irritating to your skin and allows better air circulation than tight-fitting noncotton garments. Avoid synthetic materials such as polyesters and nylons because they irritate your skin by allowing sweat and heat to accumulate. Also try to avoid rough fabrics, such as wool.

CAN I GO SUNBATHING AND SWIMMING WITH MY ECZEMA?

Don't worry. Swimming is tolerated by those whose eczema is under good control. After swimming, skin lubricants should be immediately applied before your skin becomes excessively dry and itchy. Adequate chlorination and proper pH balance are essential. Salt water may cause a burning sensation and irritate your eczematic skin. Moderate sun exposure is therapeutic.

WHAT SOAP SHOULD I USE WITH MY ECZEMA?

Ordinary soaps must be avoided because they are alkaline and remove the natural oils from your skin. Dove, Neutrogena, and Lowila are commonly recommended for the dry, itchy skin of eczema. Cetaphil Lotion may serve as a cleanser for your skin and even as a shampoo.

WHICH CREAMS ARE BEST FOR ECZEMA?

It is important to keep your skin moist. This is best accomplished with the application of creams such as Eucerin and lotions such as Cetaphil. These should be applied at least twice a day; sometimes more frequent treatment is necessary.

Creams that contain urea, such as Carmol, soften your skin. They are often very helpful and may be used frequently, but you should not use such preparations on cracked and open eczema.

Cortisone creams and ointments are helpful. Hydrocortisone cream (0.5% to 1%) is available without a prescription. Very potent cortisones are often required, but should only be used under close medical supervision. As your severe eczema clears, continue treatment with less-potent steroids, and don't forget to keep using your moisturizer. For your face, groin, and underarms, use only the weaker steroids. Carefully discuss the strengths and uses of steroid creams and ointments with your doctor. Many patients require two or three different strengths and preparations of topical cortisone for the best management of their eczema. Stronger concentrations in a large variety of prescription preparations are often required, but should only be used under close medical supervision.

Coal tar is sometimes added to steroid creams to increase the anti-inflammatory effect of cortisone. Its odor is peculiar, but tar has been used for centuries. It is very soothing.

WILL VASELINE HELP MY ECZEMA?

Under certain circumstances, yes. Prolonged bathing can dry out your skin. However, if you don't dry off completely before applying Vaseline, which is occlusive and thereby traps the moisture, then a soothing bath can instead be therapeutic.

CAN A BATH HELP MY ECZEMA?

Yes. A warm bath replenishes the water in your skin. To keep that water in your skin you need quickly to apply a moisturizer such as Eucerin or Aquaphor. The eczema is quite uncomfortable, and so the bath and warm lotion provide relief.

IS CORTISONE REALLY NECESSARY FOR MY ECZEMA?

Yes, absolutely! It is important to remember that before cortisone creams were available, most eczema never came under good control. If used with proper caution, this medicine is effective and without side effects. In severe cases, cortisone may be administered orally for a short course.

Your skin can become thin (or a new rash develop) if you use strong cortisone creams for longer than necessary. Infrequently, cortisone creams may have to be discontinued for a limited period.

ARE THERE OTHER TREATMENTS FOR ECZEMA?

Ultraviolet light B (sun lamps) and ultraviolet light A with psoralen treatments are being used effectively. Beware of excessive light treatment with children—this may result in photo-damage. Since eczema is an immune disorder, immune "modulators" such as Interferon and cyclosporin-A are being investigated.

WHAT ARE THE WHITE SPOTS ON MY ECZEMATIC CHILD'S FACE?

These usually small areas of depigmentation on the face or extremities are called *pityriasis alba*. These spots represent the mildest form of eczema. They are more apparent during summer months with sun tans, and in black children, and can be successfully treated by using 0.5% hydrocortisone topically.

SHOULD I HAVE SKIN TESTING FOR ECZEMA?

Yes. Skin testing may in fact detect allergens that contribute to your eczema condition. These allergens are most often foods, but may also be inhalants—dust mites, pollens, and molds. The skin tests are also helpful for detecting the cause of the respiratory symptoms that may accompany your eczema.

WILL ALLERGY SHOTS HELP MY ECZEMA?

Very infrequently, allergy shots will help. If your eczema is made worse during the pollen season, immunotherapy may be considered. Usually, this type of eczema is associated with pollen-induced hay fever or asthma. Allergy shots may make eczema worse and the dose may have to be reduced. In some cases, the shots may have to be discontinued.

When you are being treated with immunotherapy primarily for perennial respiratory allergies, you may initially experience a brief flareup of your eczema. This does not usually interfere with treatment.

ARE POISON OAK AND POISON IVY THE SAME?

Poison oak and poison ivy dermatitis occur primarily in North America; both give the same rash. The poison oak plant is found only in the West, however, while poison ivy grows in the East. They both produce oily *urushiols*, the oleoresins that sensitize the skin upon contact. Poison sumac falls in the same category because it also produces urushiol.

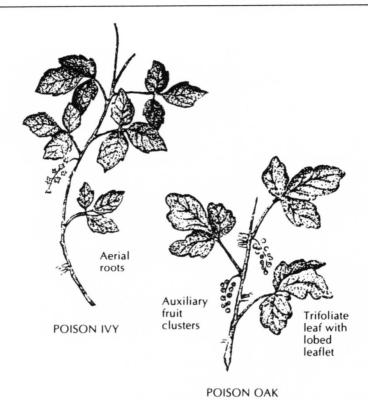

Poison ivy and poison oak.

CAN I GET POISON OAK OR POISON IVY FROM MY CLOTHING?

Yes. The oily resin will remain attached to articles of clothing until they are washed or dry-cleaned. Contact with such an adhering resin, even months later, may result in a rash.

The same thing occurs when a pet has come into contact with the plant and then carries the resin home to a loving and affectionate family.

CAN I CATCH POISON OAK FROM TOILET SEATS?

When former President Nixon and his group visited China, the toilet seats had been newly lacquered in preparation for the visiting Americans. The lacquer contained a substance very similar to the allergen of poison oak. The native Chinese were not sensitive to this substance, but many of the Americans were. The bottom line: a very embarrassing situation for all concerned.

Do Allergic People Tend to Get Poison Oak or Poison Ivy More Easily Than Nonallergies

Not really. In fact, there is evidence that those with severe allergic eczema usually cannot become sensitized to such contact allergens as poison oak.

Allergy to poison oak/ivy is different from hay fever, asthma, and the various eczemas. The urushiol contained in these plants causes a delayed skin reaction in people with sensitized white blood cells (T lymphocytes). The same type of delayed reaction is seen in allergic skin rashes to jewelry made with the most allergenic metal known, nickel. No special allergic antibodies of the IgE class are found in this kind of allergy.

How Can I Recognize the Rash of Poison Oak and Poison Ivy?

Poison oak and ivy rashes start to break out one or two days after contact with the plant. This is termed a *delayed allergic reaction.*

Your rash is initially red and slightly raised, with small "bumps," which then enlarge and become filled with a clear watery fluid. Next, your rash begins to weep and ooze. A yellowish crust is formed and soon falls off, leaving a very tender and sensitive layer of new skin exposed.

Your face, arms, hands, and genital areas are the most commonly involved sites. Severe swelling often occurs in these sensitive tissues, especially the eyelids. The rash will often trace a "streaked" pattern that was brushed by the plant. As the rash progresses, this pattern is not as obvious.

There are degrees of severity. All your affected skin is extremely itchy and uncomfortable! The poison oak or ivy rash may last up to three to four weeks without cortisone therapy.

WILL MY POISON OAK OR POISON IVY SPREAD?

Yes and no. The oily resin can remain on your fingers and under your fingernails, and thus can be spread until washed off. Likewise, the resin can remain on your boots, and unwitting further contact can cause a flareup of your rash even months later.

After touching a poison oak plant, you are likely to experience a rash first on one part of your body and, later, on another. The time it takes your rash to develop has to do with the degree of contact made with the poison oak plant, and with the thickness of your skin, which varies in different areas of your body. This "spreading" does not result from touching the *rash*, and thereby transmitting the rash from one part of your body to the other, but from spreading the urushiol resin. Often this resin is no longer present when the rash has broken out.

HOW LONG WILL MY POISON OAK OR IVY LAST?

Your poison oak or ivy will last about three to four weeks. It is important to remember that if you are taking oral cortisone (prednisone) you should continue treatment for at least ten days after the rash appears to clear up.

WHAT IS THE BEST TREATMENT FOR MY POISON OAK OR IVY?

The best treatment is cortisone. If your rash is small and not too bothersome, the cortisone may be administered as a cream or spray. If your rash is severe or involves the eyelids or genitals, however, oral prednisone is usually necessary. This should be started at very high doses for three to five days and then tapered over another eight to ten days in order to provide control over the entire course of your malady. If the prednisone is stopped sooner, there is often a severe flareup.

Antihistamines such as Benadryl or Atarax may be taken orally to help control your itching. Lotions (Calamine) can be soothing, especially if your lesions are weeping.

Should I Wash Off After Hiking to Remove the Resin Before the Rash Breaks Out?

Perhaps. If you can wash off within five or ten minutes with a non-irritating solvent such as alcohol, you may prevent the onset of the allergic reaction. The immune response, with penetration and attachment of the antigen to your skin, and thereafter reaction with the lymphocyte white cells, starts rapidly after contact. Washing an hour later is totally useless. Don't injure your skin with strong, irritating solutions.

Can I Get Poison Oak or Poison Ivy at High Altitudes?

No. These plants do not usually grow at altitudes above 5000 feet.

Can Poison Oak and Poison Ivy Be Prevented?

Allergy shots for poison oak and poison ivy, as well as an orally administered liquid preparation of the resin, were used in the past. They were not very effective, caused many complications, and we do not recommend them.

The best treatment is prevention. Avoid exposure by wearing protective clothing when you know you may be exposed to these plants. Remember to wash your exposed clothing in a hot cycle. If your clothing cannot be washed, it should be stored in a well-ventilated area for at least three weeks. Nevertheless, be aware that the poison oak resin can remain on your boots and other items, causing these reactions up to one year later. Pets who have hiked with you should be thoroughly washed before you touch them again. Protective creams that can be applied before exposure are now available. A brand currently available in pharmacies is Poison Oak-N-Ivy Armor.

The American Indians used to give their babies poison oak leaves to chew in an effort to prevent later sensitivity. Do not attempt this.

Is Poison Ivy Like Hay Fever?

Both are allergies, but the mechanisms are quite different. Hay fever, like most allergies, is caused by IgE allergy antibodies. The allergic reaction occurs within minutes of exposure to the allergen. Reactions to pollens, cats, and bee stings are called immediate hypersensitivity reactions.

In contrast, the reaction to poison ivy or poison oak becomes obvious only 24–48 hours after exposure. The body's memory for the allergic response is carried in T-lymphocyte blood cells and these cells migrate to the area where the allergenic oleoresin, urushiol, has touched the skin. The lymphocytes then secrete chemicals that cause the characteristic eruption.

There seems to be no increased incidence of poison ivy or oak allergies in hay fever sufferers. Interestingly, many with atopic dermatitis seem to be somewhat resistant to poison oak. Histamine is not involved in your poison oak rash, but antihistamines may help the itching. They do not, however, improve your rash.

WHY DO MY PIERCED EARS SWELL, BURN, AND ITCH?

Nickel is the most common metal causing allergy. Pierced ears—and other body parts—are more susceptible. The rash is a delayed skin allergy called contact dermatitis. The reaction and rash are much like poison oak. Usually, prolonged exposure is necessary to sensitize or initiate your allergy. Once sensitized, an allergic person cannot tolerate any metal containing nickel. The problem may be lessened by the use of surgical steel, high carat gold, or teflon-coated posts. Cortisone cream is usually sufficient to treat a small local reaction, but secondary infection may cause the formation of discolored matter.

A similar reaction occurs when bluejean buttons are exposed to uncovered skin. Sometimes covering the inside of the button with cloth or tape is helpful. Wrist watches and bracelets may also be a problem. Some people just cannot wear metal jewelry at all.

The diagnosis of allergy to nickel is usually based on history, but special patch tests can confirm that nickel is the culprit. A compound containing a known amount of nickel is applied to your skin and the area is observed 24 hours later. Patch testing

---

PRODUCTS THAT CAN CAUSE CONTACT DERMATITIS
- Nail polish
- Hair dyes, permanent solutions, and shampoos
- Underarm deodorants, especially antiperspirants
- Rubber or dye in shoes
- Formaldehyde in clothing and wood products
- Industrial solvents

---

is often necessary in detecting difficult-to-identify contact sensitivities and is usually done in specialized dermatology clinics.

ARE THERE OTHER PRODUCTS THAT CAN CAUSE CONTACT DERMATITIS?

Many (*see* box). Women are surprised to learn that allergy to nail polish may have caused swelling in their eyelids. After the polish is applied, these women rubbed their faces, spreading the allergen to their eyelids. The thin skin on the eyelids is particularly prone to contact dermatitis.

HOW AND WHY DO YOU GET LATEX RUBBER ALLERGY?

Latex is a natural milky sap from the tropical rubber tree. Latex is found in surgical gloves, catheters, dish washing gloves, rubber bands, balloons, dental dams, and condoms. The most common reaction is a rash called contact dermatitis similar to that from sensitization to poison oak or nickel. People allergic to avocado, bananas, and chestnuts are more prone to develop an allergy to latex.

A more recently recognized and often dramatic reaction is anaphylaxis. This may be mild to life-threatening and can include:

- Hives and generalized itching
- Asthma
- Hay fever-like symptoms
- Fatal anaphylactic shock

Exposure to latex during a surgical procedure can cause the most severe reactions. If you have experienced any reaction to latex rubber products and are scheduled for surgery, be sure to let your doctors know. All personnel need to wear nonlatex gloves. Latex catheters should not be used. Allergic patients are more susceptible to this reaction. Skin and blood tests are currently being developed to diagnose latex rubber allergy, but the history you give your doctor is the most important criterion.

5

Food Allergy

How Common Is Food Allergy?
How Does Eating Foods Cause Allergy?
What Are the Other Kinds of Food Hypersensitivity–Allergy?
Must I Eat the Food to Have an Allergic Reaction to It?
Are All Fish Reactions Allergic?
Which Are the Most Common Allergenic Foods?
What About Eating Pollen and Mold?
A Mold-Free Diet
What Is the Best Way to Diagnose Food Allergy?
Milk Elimination Diet
Corn Elimination Diet
Wheat Elimination Diet
Legume Elimination Diet
Classic Basic Elimination Diet
Are Skin Tests Helpful?
Are There Blood Tests for Food Allergies?
Have Specific Allergens Been Identified for Food Allergies?
May I Use Peanut Oil If I Am Allergic to Peanuts?
Are Food Allergy Shots Helpful? How About Sublingual Drops?
Is My Asthma Caused by Food Allergy?
Can Food Allergy Cause Hay Fever Symptoms?
Why Do I Have Allergy to Melons, Bananas, and Ragweed?
Can Foods Eaten While Exercising Cause Reactions?
*Does Alcohol Increase the Risk of a Severe Immediate Allergic
    Reaction to Foods?*
Which Foods Should Be Avoided During Infancy?
*Should I Avoid Such Allergenic Foods as Cow's Milk
    and Eggs During Pregnancy?*
*Will Breastfeeding and Delayed Introduction of Solid Foods Protect
    My Baby from Asthma and Hay Fever?*

5 Food Allergy

How Common Is Food Allergy?

Strictly speaking, *food allergy* occurs in only 2% of adults and 5 to 10% of children. The true incidence is clouded by the frequent occurrence of additional nonimmune adverse food reactions. The classic example is diarrhea from milk. Additionally, very often parents will incorrectly attribute a symptom such as hyperactivity to a food allergy.

In selected groups of patients, the incidence of documented IgE-mediated food allergy is much higher than in the general population. In children and adults with atopic dermatitis (eczema) the incidence of documented food allergy can be as high as 50%. Food allergies usually first become apparent in childhood, and although such allergic reactions are sometimes outgrown, it is important to remember that most immediate allergic reactions to peanuts, nuts, shellfish, and fish persist strongly, so that these foods can never be eaten.

How Does Eating Foods Cause Allergy?

The ingestion of foods can cause allergy in several ways. Symptoms may arise immediately or appear within several hours, and are often mediated by special IgE antibodies. These reactions to foods are the result of a sensitization process similar to that which occurs in hay fever.

Briefly, your exposure to specific food proteins causes the formation of IgE allergy antibodies. These antibodies then attach to the mast cells or basophils in your skin and in your digestive and respiratory systems. When you eat the sensitizing food again, the food's protein combines with IgE, and histamine is released. The reaction may vary greatly in severity from simply an itchy mouth (oral allergy syndrome) to generalized anaphylaxis and shock. Common symptoms include hives, angioedema, wheezing, vomiting, cramps, and diarrhea. Nasal symptoms may also be present. Almost any food can be responsible. Common sensitizers include peanuts, nuts, fish, shellfish, fresh fruits, eggs, and legumes. You may need to carry an emergency injectable-adrenalin kit and antihistamines.

> **FOOD HYPERSENSITIVITY–ALLERGY REACTIONS**
> - Milk intolerance in infants after a "stomach flu"
> - Lactase enzyme deficiency
> - Delayed onset food reactions—nasal congestion, wheezing, abdominal symptoms, middle ear infections
> - Guten protein sensitivity (wheat, oat, rye, barley)
> - Chocolate-induced headaches
> - Arthralgias—joint pain without swelling

WHAT ARE THE OTHER KINDS OF FOOD HYPERSENSITIVITY–ALLERGY?

Food hypersensitivity–allergy can also cause flareups of many conditions that are not mediated by allergic IgE antibodies. You are right when you identify a specific food as the culprit, though skin prick tests or specific IgE (RAST) blood tests fail to document these specific food hypersensitivities. Some food hypersensitivity–allergy reactions are shown in the above box.

MUST I EAT THE FOOD TO HAVE AN ALLERGIC REACTION TO IT?

No. Some with allergies to foods report that they begin to itch and develop a rash while they are preparing dinner—hives develop on their hands and arms. Surprisingly, a common offender is the juice of potatoes, and over the years, many have reported a similar reaction when peeling shrimp. The phenomenon is known as contact urticaria, and it is caused by your IgE allergy antibodies. Essentially, you have done your own skin test. If you know you suffer such a food allergy, it is essential that you wear gloves when preparing your nemesis foods.

ARE ALL FISH REACTIONS ALLERGIC?

No. A young woman, who has no allergies, was eating a "fresh" (not canned) tuna sandwich. She immediately noticed a funny sensation in her mouth and felt ill with nausea. Within 30 minutes she developed violent diarrhea and generalized flushing—her whole body turned bright red. This poisonous reaction comes from histamine in the fish, which was not quite fresh. When scromboid fish—tuna, mackerel, snapper, and roughy—are stored, their protein breaks down into chemicals including histamine. This reaction produces what is known as scromboid poisoning. Antihistamines, if available, may be helpful in overcoming the symptoms, and supportive fluids should also be taken to prevent dehydration.

Another condition sometimes confused with allergy is staphylococcal food poisoning, which results from the generation of a bacterial toxin in buffet food or picnic food not kept hot or cold enough to prevent growth of the Staphylococcus organism.

In contrast, salmonella "food poisoning" is really an *infection* caused by eating foods contaminated with the salmonella bacterium. The salmonella germ then grows in your intestine and you often develop severe nausea and diarrhea hours later. This is a particularly dangerous infection in infants and patients with immune deficiency. The infection may extend first to the blood and then to the brain. Beware, too, of raw milk, raw or undercooked eggs, and improperly handled poultry. And hamburger must always be thoroughly cooked.

WHICH ARE THE MOST COMMON ALLERGENIC FOODS?

It is no wonder that cow's milk is the most common allergenic food, since this is the food that most of us provide our newborn infants. Its products—cheese, yogurt, butter—are major food items in our diets. It is also present as the milk solids component of popular commercial bakery products, such as breads and cookies.

Egg is another common food allergen, especially the egg white. Egg whites contain a highly allergenic protein called *albumin*. In addition to egg dishes, this protein is often found in pastries and breads. Oddly enough, only rarely will an egg-sensitive individual also be allergic to chicken.

Of the cereal grains, the most common offenders are wheat and corn. These potential food allergens should be introduced into an infant's diet slowly and then only after rice and oats have been tolerated.

Legumes, for example, peanuts, are often associated with immediate allergic reactions. Soybeans, another legume, are also allergenic and are growing in popularity in our diets. More soybean allergies are expected in the near future. Did you know that licorice is also a legume, as are beans, peas, alfalfa, lentils, and bean sprouts.

Seafoods, especially shellfish, are notoriously well known for their severe immediate allergic reactions. Some sensitive individuals actually experience asthma attacks simply by smelling the odor of fish or shellfish.

Chocolate may cause headaches and skin rashes. Cola drinks and cocoa-containing foods should also be avoided in chocolate-sensitive individuals.

WHAT ABOUT EATING POLLEN AND MOLD?

Bee pollen is really plant pollen, mainly the pollen of flowers, as well as bee body parts. It is an outrageously expensive form of protein. If you are sensitive to pollens or to bees, you can develop a severe, life-threatening reaction when you eat bee pollen. A patient in Walnut Creek, California, expected a burst of energy after ingesting her pollen, but instead went into anaphylactic shock with a precipitous drop in blood pressure. Fortunately, she was near an Emergency Room and survived.

If you are sensitive to mold spores and have asthma, your symptoms may flareup after you ingest foods with high mold content. Such foods include: cheese, yogurt, mushrooms, and even soy sauce. A three-week trial elimination diet and a subsequent challenge may be helpful.

A MOLD-FREE DIET

Foods eliminated:
- Cheeses of all types (including cottage cheese), sour cream, buttermilk, sour milk, yogurt
- Mushrooms, soy sauce
- Beer, wine
- Cider
- Vinegar foods—pickles, mayonnaise, ketchup, relish, olives, sauerkraut

- Pickled and smoked meats—sausage, hot dogs, pastrami, tongue
- Sour breads, pumpernickel, fresh rolls, coffee cakes, and other foods with high yeast content
- Dried fruit, including raisins
- Canned tomatoes and tomato sauce (spaghetti, pizza)
- Canned juices—especially apple and tomato
- Cantaloupe
- Peanuts
- Previously ground meat and opened canned foods

WHAT IS THE BEST WAY TO DIAGNOSE FOOD ALLERGY?

The most reliable method of diagnosing suspect nonimmediate food allergy is the trial elimination diet. If a limited number of selected foods are properly eliminated for two to three weeks, the allergen is most often identified. The return of the symptoms after subsequent challenges may help to confirm the diagnosis. However, most patients are not too anxious to make themselves sick again after achieving a significant remission. Such challenges are really only necessary when the improvement is not clear-cut and remains questionable. A subsequent challenge should never be attempted when the initial food reaction is immediate and life-threatening.

If you would like to uncover a possible allergy to foods such as milk, wheat, corn, and legumes, the following diets may prove helpful.

MILK ELIMINATION DIET

Foods eliminated:
- Liquid milk or cream, whether used as a drink, on cereal, on fruit, or elsewhere
- Evaporated milk, dried milk, skimmed milk,* goat's milk
- Cottage cheese and all other cheese classes; yogurt, custard, junket

*Skimmed milk is lower in fat, but contains a large amount of the allergenic protein.

- Ice cream and sherbet (sherbet contains as much milk protein as ice cream)
- Pancakes and waffles made with milk (many mixes contain dried milk and should not be used)

OK to eat:
- All foods that are not specifically eliminated above may be eaten; all meats, vegetables, and fruits are allowed.

The following foods have traces of milk solids and may be tolerated by less sensitive milk allergic patients:

- Bakery products, including bread, rolls, cookies, cakes and pies, butter and margarine.
- Mocha Mix and Eden Soy are cream substitutes; use them on cereals and for cooking (pancakes and waffles); they may be too rich to be used as a drink, but some allergics drink them after adding water.
- Soybean milks can be substituted for cow's milk in infants; Nutramigen, Pregestimil, and Alimentum are good substitutes when used with a nipple bottle—their odors tend to be very unpleasant. Soybean milks can also be substituted.
- Sorbets and granitas are usually milk-free; check the recipe.

If milk elimination is to be continued after this trial diet, a calcium substitute may be used in children.

CORN ELIMINATION DIET

Some of the following foods need not be eliminated entirely. Exceptions and substitutes are listed under "OK to Use" for those items marked with an asterisk (*).

Foods eliminated:

Corn syrup:
- Canned fruits and nectars
- Peanut butter*
- Mayonnaise*
- Sweetened cereals
- Mocha Mix and Coffee Rich
- Jams and jellies*
- Ice cream*
- Catsup
- Pancake syrup*
- Candies

Corn cereal:
- Fresh, canned, frozen corn
- Hominy grits

- Popcorn
- Fritos
- Cornmeal
- Mexican food

- Corn flakes
- Cheerios
- Beer

Corn starch:
- Chinese food (not all)
- Prepared gravies and soups

- Prepared bakery products
- Powdered sugar

Corn meal and corn flour:
- Corn bread
- Corn muffins

- Pancake and waffle mixes
- Fish sticks

Corn oil:
- Mazola*
- Potato chips*

- Margarine
- Salad oil and dressing

OK to eat:
- Best Foods mayonnaise
- Hellman's mayonnaise
- Homemade jams and jellies
- Pure maple syrup
- Spry, Crisco, Wesson Oil
- Ice cream made without corn sweetener

- Olive oil
- Natural peanut butter
- Potato chips without corn oil

- Arrowroot (for thickening)

WHEAT ELIMINATION DIET

Foods eliminated:
- Ordinary flour: in general, *all* regular bakery goods
- Bread: crackers, buns, biscuits, graham crackers, wafers, pancakes, cones, wheat matzos, macaroons, cakes, cookies, dumplings, doughnuts, pretzels, pie crust, rolls, wheat germ, many cereals
- Pasta and noodles: macaroni, spaghetti, vermicelli, ravioli
- Foods with cereal or bread fillers: stuffing, gravy, chili, cream sauces, meatloaf, fried food coatings
- Postum

OK to eat:
- Ry-Krisp
- Rice Krispies
- Cream of Rice
- Oatmeal
- Tapioca
- Potato, rice, and soy flour
- Grainless mix

Wheat- and gluten-free products can be purchased at reliable health food stores.

LEGUME ELIMINATION DIET

Foods eliminated:
- Beans
- Peas
- Soybean
- Peanuts
- Licorice
- Tragacanth (vegetable gum)

Ideally, only one food should be tested at a time.

CLASSIC BASIC ELIMINATION DIET

On rare occasions the basic elimination diet is necessary and can be very helpful. Some of the following foods cover most, but not all, *hidden* allergies.

Foods eliminated:
- Milk
- Chocolate and cola beverages
- Egg
- Citrus fruits (orange, lemon, grapefruit)
- Legumes
- Tomato
- Corn
- Wheat
- Rice
- Oats
- Barley
- Rye
- Millet
- Food colors and preservatives
- Cinnamon

OK to eat:
- Apple (peeled), apple juice, applesauce
- Banana, pear
- Grape, grape juice, vinegar, raisin
- Pineapple, pineapple juice
- Almond, apricot, cherry, peach, plum, prune
- Cranberry, blueberry, raspberry, blackberry
- Loganberry, strawberry, gooseberry
- Sugar (maple, brown, white)
- Clove
- Mint
- Tea
- Hazel nut, wintergreen
- Cashew nut
- Brazil nut
- Pine nut
- Olive
- Avocado
- Cucumber, pickles, squash, pumpkin,

- Fig
- Persimmon
- Rhubarb, buckwheat
- Coconut, date
- Papaya
- Vanilla
- Ginger, arrowroot
- Artichoke, lettuce
- Beet, spinach, swiss chard
- Cauliflower
- Fish
- Asparagus, onion
- Green pepper, red pepper

cantaloupe, melons
- Mushroom
- Sweet potato
- Radish, turnip,
  broccoli, cabbage
  brussel sprouts,
  Chinese cabbage,
  collards, kale
- Carrot, celery
- Clams, abalone,
  scallops, oysters,
  shrimp, lobster
- Chicken, turkey, lamb

Remember, any cheating or mistakes will invalidate the test diet. Keep a careful record of your symptoms prior to and during the trial period. A current illness, such as a respiratory infection, will, of course, interfere with the test.

ARE SKIN TESTS HELPFUL?

Skin tests for foods using the scratch method may provide some help with diagnosis. They can be misleading for delayed-onset reactions and must be interpreted in the light of clinical history: the age of onset of symptoms, the types of foods in the diet, and, most important, the results of a trial elimination diet.

Skin tests are useful in the diagnosis of immediate reactions. Since systemic allergic reactions can occur from the testing itself, this procedure should be carefully undertaken only after a thorough history. When a specific food is suspected as the cause of a severe reaction, your physician should either begin testing with diluted test material or order a blood test.

Routine skin testing for a large number of foods is rarely necessary or helpful. Be skeptical if the testing of 30 or more foods is suggested.

Very often skin tests are truly positive, indicating that you have IgE antibodies to certain foods though, in fact, you know you can eat these foods with impunity. At the moment, we simply don't know why some people with allergy skin-test antibodies to foods can eat those foods while others suffer disastrous consequences. For example, in our practices we may see a patient with hay fever or hives, but no food allergy symptoms. If we carry out ten skin tests for food allergy, we may obtain a positive reaction for peanuts or eggs, and upon questioning find that the presumably allergic patient eats peanuts and eggs daily without problems. A relevant skin test must always be correlated with a positive clinical history.

If you suspect you are experiencing an allergic reaction to an unusual food or spice such as cumin, annatto, or kiwi, your allergist will need to prepare special skin test reagents because they are simply not always commercially available.

ARE THERE BLOOD TESTS FOR FOOD ALLERGIES?

Yes. The RAST blood tests, which detect the same IgE food antibodies as do the skin tests. They are most helpful in confirming and quantitating the allergies that cause severe, immediate reactions to such specific foods, as peanuts and fish. Although the cause of your allergic symptoms may seem obvious, confirmation with RAST is important; after all, you want to make sure that you don't rule a food out of your diet unnecessarily. Additionally, it may be useful to compare the level of your allergic sensitivity to that food in future years.

For patients with life-threatening reactions to foods, the RAST test is simpler, and sometimes safer, than tedious skin testing using serial dilutions. Sometimes, too, the RAST test may be negative when an allergic sensitivity is truly present; in this case such serial-dilution skin testing is necessary and will give the most reliable results. However, RAST tests are not available for all food allergens.

When properly performed, RAST testing can provide you and your physician with important information. Not all techniques and laboratories are reliable, and quality control is most important. As with skin testing, laboratory results must be carefully interpreted in the light of your clinical history.

HAVE SPECIFIC ALLERGENS BEEN IDENTIFIED FOR FOOD ALLERGIES?

Yes, but only for a limited number of foods. The cow's milk protein allergens are:

- Casein
- Whey proteins
    beta-lactoglobulin
    alpha-lactalbumin
- Bovine serum albumin
- Bovine serum gamma globulin

When cow's milk is separated into curds and whey, the predominant curd protein is casein, which is made into cheese; whey is the odoriferous liquid that contains all the other allergenic proteins. The whey protein, beta-lactoglobulin, is the most potent allergenic substance in milk. Whey is commonly used in food processing, especially in bakery goods. Casein is also present in goat's milk, so the latter is not always an adequate substitute for cow's milk.

The protein, Allergen M, has been identified as the allergen in codfish. The proteins in egg that cause allergy are found in the egg white and include ovalbumin, ovomucoid, and ovotransferrin. Though many who are allergic to eggs are able to eat egg yolk, this can be dangerous since particles of egg white may adhere. Specific allergens have also been identified for soybean (soybean trypsin inhibitor), shrimp (Peni I), and two separate allergens for the most dangerous allergenic food, peanuts (Ara h I and II).

MAY I USE PEANUT OIL IF I AM ALLERGIC TO PEANUTS?

Studies have shown that peanut oil is safe. Pure peanut oil is an unsaturated fat that does not contain the peanut allergens, Ara h I and II. Enjoy your potato chips and your Chinese stir-fry foods prepared in peanut oil. All other peanut products will cause your allergies to flare up and must be strictly avoided if you are sensitive. Sunflower oil has also been studied and is tolerated by many who are allergic to sunflower seeds. The explanation is that the allergenic protein substance is not soluble in oil.

ARE FOOD ALLERGY SHOTS HELPFUL? HOW ABOUT SUBLINGUAL DROPS?

Food allergy shots and sublingual drops have not been demonstrated to be helpful when controlled studies are carried out. In fact, though testimonies from many allergics exist to suggest the efficacy of food shots, and even of food drops placed under the tongue, these forms of treatment remain controversial and are potentially dangerous and life-threatening. Although sublingual drops would not be expected to work, active research to develop an effective form of allergy shots for peanuts has been carried out. Again, food shots should currently only be taken within experimental programs offered in qualified research centers. Today the only reliable treatment for food allergy remains elimination.

IS MY ASTHMA CAUSED BY FOOD ALLERGY?

If you suffer asthma accompanied by severe wheezing and intermittent coughing with bronchospasm, your allergy specialist will want to take a thorough medical history along with your physical examination. Do not blame the asthma of infancy and childhood on foods without investigating other causes. Necessary studies you may be asked to permit include a chest X-ray, breathing tests for pulmonary function, and skin testing. Other tests that may be strongly recommended are sinus X-rays, a sweat test, blood tests, and sputum studies for infections and eosinophils. Remember, not all that wheezes is asthma—and not all asthma is allergy.

If all these tests are negative, your allergist may consider a hidden food allergy. Milk and grains (especially corn and wheat) will sometimes be responsible for allergic manifestations, even with a negative skin test. A trial elimination diet for two to three weeks may identify a suspect food and thus lead to improvement of your asthma.

CAN FOOD ALLERGY CAUSE HAY FEVER SYMPTOMS?

If you are allergic to foods as well as pollens, you may be exquisitely sensitive to even small amounts of food during the pollen season. Your specific food elimination diet must be very strict without any "slip-ups." At other times of the year, a less rigid diet may be tolerated and your perennial symptoms will usually remain under adequate control. If you are allergic to milk and grass, you may have more trouble with milk during the peak grass pollen season.

Only after eliminating inhalant allergies and nonallergic rhinitis as well as various other factors such as infections, side effects to your medicines, and such conditions as pregnancy, should you consider food allergies as causes of your hay fever-type symptoms. With immediate allergic reactions, such as that to peanuts, the cause is usually obvious and there are associated eye, throat, or skin reactions. If this is not the case, then a carefully selected trial elimination diet and subsequent challenge may clearly demonstrate a food to be the cause of your respiratory allergic symptoms.

WHY DO I HAVE ALLERGIES TO MELONS, BANANAS, AND RAGWEED?

If you are sensitive to certain airborne allergens, you can be more sensitive to specific foods because there are cross-reactive allergens that have similar chemical configurations:

- Ragweed: melons, bananas, and camomile tea
- Mugwort weed pollen: celery
- Birch pollen: apple, carrot, and hazelnut
- Latex rubber (often airborne particles): banana, avocado, chestnut

CAN FOODS EATEN WHILE EXERCISING CAUSE REACTIONS?

Exercise 30 minutes to two hours after the ingestion of specific foods has been shown to cause generalized hives, wheezing, and anaphylactic shock in some who suffer food allergies. Celery (an unlikely suspect) and shrimp were initially reported, and many other foods may also be responsible. With this condition, your skin test results are positive, and you are of course always allergic, but the allergic reaction occurs only when exercise follows ingestion of that specific food. Your treatment is simply to avoid that combination of food and exercise. And you should also keep adrenalin and antihistamines handy.

DOES ALCOHOL INCREASE THE RISK OF A SEVERE IMMEDIATE ALLERGIC REACTION TO FOODS?

Yes. When you are at a party and have a few drinks, you will be relaxed and not concentrating on what is on the *hors d'oeuvres* tray. If you are sensitive to certain nuts or to sesame seeds, this is the most frequent "set-up" for a severe, life-threatening allergic reaction to those nuts or the sesame seeds that may be part of the snacks. Moreover, some allergists have suggested that alcohol facilitates the body's rapid absorption of food allergens, accelerating your allergic reactions. Beware! You cannot let your guard down.

WHICH FOODS SHOULD BE AVOIDED DURING INFANCY?

Exclusive breastfeeding for the first six months provides your infant with the best food, especially when that child is allergy-prone. Mothers who breastfeed should avoid such allergenic foods as peanuts, fish, cow's milk, and eggs. If breastfeeding is not possible, predigested milk products—protein hydrolysates such as Nutramigen, Pregestimil, and Alimentum—may be used. Soybean formulas have been successfully used for decades; however, a significant number of infants who are allergic to milk may also become allergic to soybean. Changes in formula can be burdensome for your infant as well as for you, but an ounce of prevention is worth eight ounces of cure.

If your infant is highly allergic to milk, showing such immediate reactions as hives and anaphylaxis, it may be reacting even to such protein hydrolysates as Nutramigen as well as to the newer hypoallergenic formulas such as Good Start. These special formulas contain enough "look-alike" milk proteins to cause dangerous and sometimes fatal reactions in highly sensitive, milk allergic infants. Cow's milk allergy occurs in 1% of infants in the general population, and obviously in a significantly higher percentage of infants from allergic parents.

SHOULD I AVOID SUCH ALLERGENIC FOODS AS COW'S MILK AND EGGS DURING PREGNANCY?

Generally, no. You should not follow special allergy-avoidance diets during pregnancy. These diets do not have any beneficial effect on your baby's possible future development of allergy. In fact, the restriction of nutritious foods can be harmful for both mother and child. Nevertheless, some prudence is advised—eating excessive amounts of highly allergenic foods such as eggs and peanuts can cause your baby to be born with allergies to these foods. Your child might then experience a severe reaction on the very first exposure to them.

WILL BREASTFEEDING AND DELAYED INTRODUCTION OF SOLID FOODS PROTECT MY BABY FROM ASTHMA AND HAY FEVER?

Possibly. Though feeding precautions can protect against the inception of food allergy and eczema, viral infections are the most important cause of asthma in the first years of life.

WHAT FOODS SHOULD I INTRODUCE FIRST TO MY BABY?

Breast milk is highly nutritious and is the recommended food for your infant. Iron, fluoride, and vitamins A, C, and D are the only supplements that may be necessary for complete nutrition of your breastfed baby for the first year of its life. Thereafter, the introduction of selected allergy-causing foods should be gradual. No solid foods should be introduced into your baby's diet until the age of four to six months, especially if the baby is premature. A premature digestive tract will allow the absorption of the larger allergenic food molecules and thus may allow the induction of an allergic reaction in your child. Each new food should be added to your baby's diet at two-week intervals so that, should any adverse food reaction occur, that food can be easily identified and removed from its diet.

If your infant is allergy-prone, breast milk should be continued as long as possible. Soy milk may be introduced cautiously at six months, and cow's milk after one year of age. Solid foods should be delayed for at least six months; then they should be started with cereals. As for cereals, rice and oats are the least allergenic and should be introduced before wheat and corn. Eggs should not be added to your child's diet until after the age of one year.

SHOULD I BREASTFEED?

Yes. The best food for your normal newborn baby is breast milk. Although commercially prepared milk formulas are easily available and often are more convenient to feed, your breast milk is superior. It is not allergenic, has higher bioavailability for zinc, iron, and other minerals, and is far more economical.

Breast milk provides your infant the major advantage of immunologic protection against food allergies and invading infectious organisms. It contains naturally occurring IgA antibodies that protect the infant's immature gastrointestinal system. Commercial formulas do not contain these protective IgA antibodies.

DOESN'T EVERYBODY NEED MILK?

"One man's food is another man's poison." This old saying is especially true about milk. Most conventional milk formulas are cow's milk. Some infants become sick by developing either allergy or intolerance to it.

Milk proteins can easily sensitize the allergy-prone infant, and, once sensitized, your child may develop eczema, hay fever symptoms with nasal congestion and discharge, middle ear infections, asthma with coughing and wheezing, and gastrointestinal symptoms—diarrhea. Your child can become seriously ill and hospitalization sometimes may be necessary.

Milk intolerance is even more common. This occurs as a result of an enzymatic deficiency in the intestines. The enzyme *lactase* is necessary to metabolize the lactose sugar that is present in cow's milk. Those who are deficient in this enzyme would experience vomiting, bloating, cramps, and diarrhea after milk ingestion. Among Asians and blacks, more than 70% have developed lactase deficiency by the time they reach adulthood. When powdered milk was recently sent to one underdeveloped country, the local black population used it for wall paint, recognizing that milk invariably would induce diarrhea when they drank it. Lactase supplements (Lactaid) may be taken orally or added to milk to help eliminate this problem.

When allergy problems are caused by cow's milk during infancy, the milk is often replaced by a soy formula. Sensitization to soy may also then occur, and other types of milk (Nutramigen, Pregestimil, Alimentum) are good alternatives. As your infant's diet expands to include solids, milk becomes less important as a food source.

You can totally eliminate milk from your child's diet once it begins to eat adequate amounts of meat and vegetables; however, calcium and vitamin D may not always be adequately supplied in the diet of a nonmilk-drinking child. You can obtain calcium-fortified vitamin D without a prescription. And whenever making homemade soups, throw the bones in!

How About Poi as a Milk Substitute?

In the South Seas, poi is used as a milk substitute. Derived from the taro root, it provides a hearty food substance with minimal allergic potential.

Is Colitis an Allergy?

In some individuals, this may well be an allergic disease, although the immunological mechanisms have not yet been demonstrated. Some forms of colitis improve with the elimination of certain foods. The first food you should eliminate for a trial period is milk; this most frequently gives the best results. Certain drugs, such as ampicillin, may also cause colitis. Gluten-containing grains such as wheat, oats, rye, and barley may affect the small intestine and result in a serious malabsorption problem called *celiac disease* (in children) and nontropical sprue (in adults). Celiac disease is an autoimmune disease in which your own antibodies attack the cells of your intestines. This disease is triggered by gluten, which must be eliminated from your diet. Gluten is also associated with a severe, rare skin problem—dermatitis herpetiformis.

CAN YOU SUGGEST ANY SUBSTITUTES FOR THE PRINCIPAL ALLERGY-INDUCING FOODS?

Cow's milk: Soy is the most frequently used substitute. Beware, however, since the glycoprotein of soybean may also be allergenic. Excellent substitutes are Nutramigen, Pregestimil, and Alimentum.

Corn and wheat: Various grains, such as rice, barley, and rye, may be substituted for corn and wheat. Read labels carefully since few breads are made without wheat. Buckwheat is a grain unrelated to such cereal grasses as corn, wheat, rice, and oats; you may use it as a wheat substitute, though you can't make bread from it. Beware, since buckwheat itself may be a potent allergen.

Chocolate: Carob is a good substitute for chocolate but, again, remember that carob itself is a legume related to peas, beans, and soybeans, and thus also capable of producing allergic reactions.

Citrus: Other fruit juices and nectars may be adequate substitutes. Remember that most nectars you buy contain 25% corn syrup, something that is not necessarily mentioned on the label.

Nuts and peanuts: There are no substitutes for nuts and peanuts. These are often found in minute quantities in such bakery products as cookies and muffins. An extremely sensitive person should not trust any commercial bakery product even if the label does not mention nuts. You can only be sure about the cookies you bake in your own oven. Walnut-flavored peanuts are becoming popular, so do not be deceived if you are sensitive to peanuts.

Fish: It is not difficult to substitute meat for fish. However, severe life-threatening reactions have occurred even when patients who are allergic to fish are exposed to the odors of this food. If you are allergic to fish, beware of walking into a house or restaurant where fish is being cooked.

It is wise to use a substitute sparingly; otherwise, you may develop sensitivity to the new food. Don't jump from the frying pan into the fire.

Elimination diets for some of the more allergenic foods can be found earlier in this chapter. The following are recipes that are available:

Wheat, Milk and Egg-Free Recipes (free)

Quaker Oats Company
Consumer Response Group
PO Box 049001, Suite 11-3
Chicago, Illinois 60604-9001
Phone: 312-222-7843

Diets Unlimited for Limited Diets ($14.95)

Allergy/Asthma Information Association
65 Tromley Drive, Suite 10
Etobicoke, Ontario M9B5Y7
Canada
Phone: 416-244-9312

Food Sensitivity (includes cooking with Isomil) ($2.00)

Ross Laboratories
Department L-1120
Columbus, Ohio 43260
Phone: 800-227-5767

The Allergy Cookbook and Food-Buying Guide

by Pamela P. Nonken and S. Roger Hirsh, MD
Available at bookstores

Cooking for People with Food Allergies ($1.50)

USDA HG246 March 21, 1933
Superintendent of Documents
PO Box 371954
Pittsburgh, PA 15250-7954

IF I HAVE A FOOD ALLERGY, WILL OTHER FOODS IN THE SAME FAMILY CAUSE A REACTION?

This is usually not a problem. Nevertheless, there is the possibility that other botanically related foods may cause reactions. The following tables may serve as a guide.

FOOD PLANT FAMILIES

Family	Related plants	Family	Related plants
Apple	Apple	Myrtle	Allspice
	Loquat		Chilian guava
	Pear		Clove
Banana	Chestnut		Guava
Birch	Filbert	Nightshade	Bell pepper
	Hazelnut		Cayenne pepper
Buckwheat	Dock		Chili
	Rhubarb		Eggplant
Cashew	Mango	(Nightshade)	Potato
	Pistachio		Strawberry tomato
Citrus	Citron		Tomato
	Grapefruit		Tree tomato
	Kumquat	Nutmeg	Mace
	Lemon	Olive	Jasmine
	Lime		Manna
	Orange	Orchid	Salep
	Tangelo		Vanilla
	Tangerine	Palm	Cabbage palm
Cocoa	Coca leaf		Coconut
	Chocolate		Date
	Cola		Oil palm
	Karraya	Parsely	Anise
Ebony	Persimmon		Black cumin
Fungus	Morell		Caraway seed
	Mushroom		Carrot
	Truffle		Celery
Ginger	Turmeric		and celeriac
Goosefoot	Beet		Coriander
	Lamb's quarters		Cumin
	Spinach		Dill
	Swiss chard		Fennel
Gourd	Cantaloupe		Star anise

(continued)

FOOD PLANT FAMILIES *(CONTINUED)*

Family	Related plants	Family	Related plants
	Chinese watermelon		Sweet cicily
			Sweet fennel
	Cucumber	Passionflower	Passion fruit
	Gherkin	Pea (legume)	Alfalfa
	Pumpkin		Black-eyed pea, cowpea
	Summer squash		
Grape	American grape		Carob bean
	European grape		Chick pea
Grass	Bamboo		Clovers
	Barley		Common bean
(Grass)	Canary grass	*(Pea)*	(navy, kidney, pinto, string)
	Citronella		
	Corn		Jack bean
	Millet		Lentil
	Oats		Licorice
	Popcorn		Mesquite
	Rice		Peanut
	Rye		Tamarind
	Sorghum and milo		Tragacanth
		Pine	Juniper
	Sugar cane		Pinyon nut
	Wheat	Plum	Almond
	Wild rice		Apricot
Heather	Black huckleberry		Cherry
	Blueberry		Peach, nectarine
	Cranberry		Prune
Laurel	Avocado		Sloe
	Bay leaf		Wild cherry
	Cinnamon	Poppy	Poppyseed
	Sassafras	Protea	Macadamia nut
Lily	Asparagus	Rose	Black raspberry
	Chives		Boysenberry, dewberry, loganberry
	Garlic		
	Leek		
	Onion		Red raspberry
	Sarsaparilla		Strawberry
	Shallot	Saxifrage	Currant
Madder	Black guava	Senna	Tamarind
	Coffee	Spurge	Tapioca

(continued)

FOOD PLANT FAMILIES *(CONTINUED)*

Family	Related plants	Family	Related plants
Mallow	Cottonseed	Sunflower	Artichoke
	Durian	(aster)	Camomile
	Okra		Chicory
Mimosa	Acacia		Dandelion
	Basil		Endive
(Mimosa)	Catnip	*(Sunflower)*	Jerusalem
	Common mint		artichoke
	Curled mint		Safflower
	Lavender		Lettuce
	Marjoram		Sunflower seed
	Oregano		Tarragon
	Peppermint	Walnut	Butternut
	Sage		Hickory nut
	Savory		Pecan
	Spearmint		
	Spike lavender		
	Thyme		
Morning glory	Sweet potato		
Mulberry	Breadfruit		
	Fig		
	Hop		
Mustard	Broccoli		
	Brussels sprouts		
	Cabbage		
	Chinese cabbage		
	Collards and kale		
	Garden cress		
	Horseradish		
	Kohlrabi		
	Radish		
	Rape		
	Rutabaga		
	Sea kale		
	Turnip		
	Watercress		

OUTLINE OF ANIMAL FOODS

Amphibians	Frogs	Fish	Perch
Birds	Duck		Flounder,
	Goose		halibut
	Dove, squab		Grayling,
	Turkeys		red salmon,
	Guinea fowl		pink salmon,
	Partridge		whitefish
	and quail		Croaker, drum,
	Chicken,		redfish,
	guinea fowl,		squeteague,
	pheasant		weakfish
Crustaceans	Crayfish		Bonito, mackerel,
	Crabs		tuna
	Shrimp		Grouper, white bass,
	Lobsters		rock fish
	Prawns		Bullhead, catfish
Fish	Sturgeon		Sole
	Smelts		Porgy, red snapper
	Eel		Anchovy
	Pompano		Swordfish
	Black bass,	Mammals	Cow, goat, sheep
	crappie,		Deer
	sunfish,		Hare, rabbit
	herring,		Squirrel
	menhaden,		Pig
	sardine,	Mollusks	Cockle
	shad, sprat		Abalone
	Carp, chub		Snail
	Muskellunge,		Periwinkle
	pickerel, pike		Clam
	Cod, haddock,		Mussel
	pollack,		Octopus
	whiting		Oyster
	Hake		Scallon
	Mullet		Squid

6

Insect Allergy

How Do Insects Cause Allergy?

Some insects cause allergies by biting or stinging; others cause severe allergic reactions when their body parts or feces are inhaled. Bees, ants, kissing bugs, fleas, and mosquitoes are part of the first group. The second group consists of cockroaches, crickets, caddis fly, May fly, and the insect-like house dust mites.

Insect prevalence depends a great deal on geographic factors. The caddis and May flies are common severe problems in the Great Lakes region. Urban dwellers experience more house dust mite and cockroach allergy, whereas rural populations are more exposed to bees and yellow jackets (Hymenoptera). One-half percent of the general population experiences severe allergic anaphylactic reactions to bee stings. The most likely victim of a bee sting is a young man under age 20, but this can certainly can occur in older patients. Local reactions can be very mild, with itching and swelling, to massive swelling of an entire arm or leg occuring in 5% of the general population.

How About House Dust Mites?

One of the most important allergy components of house dust is the house dust mite, *Dermatophagoides*. This "insect" is 0.3 millimeters in length and barely visible without a microscope. Mites have eight legs (imagine how tiny) and are arachnoids, like spiders. With appropriate humidity and temperature during certain seasons, there is marked proliferation with an increased concentration of this insect. San Francisco and London provide favorable climates.

The house dust mite feeds on animal materials with high protein content, especially human dander; thus the name *Dermatophagoides*, "skin eater." The dust mite also feeds on mold. It has been found and studied in Europe, America, and the Far East and is the allergen that makes house dust antigenically similar in these distant geographic locations. The specific antigen of the mite is found in its feces and is, in fact, a digestive enzyme.

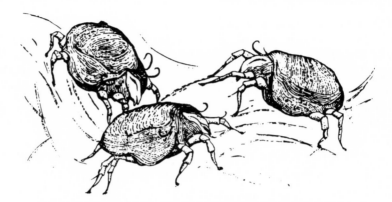

House dust mites (magnified more than 200 times).

CAN I BE ALLERGIC TO FLEA BITES?

Yes. Many allergics develop large and extremely itchy local reactions to flea bites, though it often appears that only one or two family members are being bitten. Actually, the 20 species of fleas that bite people show no discretion—they bite everyone. Like mosquitoes, they are bloodsuckers and deposit an anticoagulant in the skin. Only the sensitive individual develops a local allergic reaction to this anticoagulant. The site itches and the reaction consists of redness, swelling, tiny to large blisters, or large, fixed hives. Don't be fooled because no one else in the family is affected. They are simply fortunate not to be allergic. The most common site of reaction is the ankle, which is close to the carpet where the fleas frolic. The itch can be intense and by the time we see the flea-bitten allergics, they have often developed secondary infections from scratching. Pets contribute to the problem by providing a source of warm blood for fleas. When the pet is out, you are the target. Fleas are also found in sandboxes and at the beach. In areas where fleas are prevalent, repeated flea bites may actually desensitize you; that is, the fleas continue to bite but the allergic reaction slowly subsides.

WILL VITAMIN B-1 (THIAMINE) HELP MY FLEA BITES?

Folklore say yes. An over-the-counter preparation, thiamine, somehow elicits a noxious odor from the skin that repels fleas. Also, you can add flea bites to the unending list of ailments that seem to be treatable by the remedy, garlic. You can reduce the number of fleas, and hence your bites, by repeated vacuuming and steam cleaning of carpets. Flea collars and insecticide fogs are helpful.

WHERE IS COCKROACH ALLERGY A PROBLEM?

New York City is probably the cockroach capital of the world! These insects are everywhere, however, and are extremely hardy. A cockroach can survive on a drop of water for a year. Eight different species of cockroaches are frequently found indoors. Some species are hardier than others. They have been on this planet for millions of years and are unlikely to disappear. You need only get up in the morning, turn on the kitchen light, and watch them scatter.

When they die or are exterminated, cockroaches slowly dry out and are pulverized, eventually creating a strong airborne allergen. Their feces are also allergenic. This explains the special advantage of the cockroach motel; as the ad says, they check in, but they don't check out. Thus you also throw away the allergen their carcasses and feces would otherwise leave in your environment. Sensitized allergics may develop both acute and chronic asthma, as well as nasal allergy symptoms, in response to cockroach allergens.

WHY DOES THE FARMER AWAKEN WITH HIVES?

In rural areas there exists a romantic bug that "kisses" its victims at night. The *Triotoma protracta* (kissing bug) creeps into bed and painlessly bites its victim, who is rudely awakened by intense itching. Untreated, the reaction can progress to typical anaphylaxis with hives, troubled breathing, and even shock.

One victim living in a wooded "suburban" area awoke at 4:30 AM with tingling and pain in his palms. The tingling then spread to his crotch and soles, and over the next few minutes the heat and tingling increased throughout his entire body. This reaction had happened before, and he sent his wife to the car for his epinephrine kit, injected the epinephrine, and chewed a 4 milligram tablet of Chlor-Trimeton. By 5:30 AM he felt fine and went out for his morning run. After injecting the epinephrine he and his wife searched the bedclothes as had been suggested by the allergist during his last visit, when the EpiPen had been prescribed. Sure enough, they found the dark brown, one inch bug later identified as *Triatoma protracta*. Positive skin tests for kissing bug saliva clinched the diagnosis. Since the reaction can be fatal and comes without warning, desensitization with allergy shots is recommended and helpful. Our victim now keeps an adrenalin kit permanently at his bedside.

WHAT ARE FIRE ANTS?

Fire ants (*Hymenoptera*) are close relatives of the bees and vespids, are found in the southern United States, and live in mounds in the ground. Fire ants first bite the victim with their jaws, then pivot their bodies, inflicting multiple stings. Both the bites and the stings are excruciatingly painful. Long-lasting local reactions and minute areas of dead skin may result. As with bees, the venom can cause severe, potentially fatal anaphylactic reactions. Allergy shots are recommended in certain cases of sensitization.

HOW IS INSECT STING ALLERGY DIAGNOSED?

The most important diagnostic tool is a good medical history. If you are stung by an insect and develop hives on other areas of the body, or have other systemic signs or symptoms such as trouble breathing, generalized itching, or swelling of the tongue and throat, or go into anaphylactic shock—you have an allergy to that insect.

Skin testing with venom for the various insects will identify and confirm your specific sensitivity. Blood tests (RAST) may also be done as part of your evaluation. The skin test is more sensitive than the blood test, and is necessary for diagnosis and treatment with venom injections. The blood test alone may miss your sensitivity.

WILL MY INSECT ALLERGY REACTIONS BECOME MORE SEVERE?

Local reactions do not generally progress to systemic allergic reactions; however, if you have suffered a true allergic systemic or generalized reaction to an insect sting, it is likely that this may happen again. Your immune system becomes more sensitive, so that more IgE allergic antibodies are produced.

On the other hand, multiple stings will sometimes actually desensitize you through a mechanism similar to that which gives allergy shots their efficacy. This sometimes occurs in allergic beekeepers; repeated stings, however, are potentially fatal.

CAN ALLERGY TO INSECT STING BE CURED?

Yes. You can receive allergy shots for bee sting and fire ant allergy, as well as allergy to May fly, caddis fly, and kissing bugs. This treatment will desensitize you so that you will not react to subsequent stings. Ninety-five percent of allergics who receive immunotherapy with bee venom are cured while they are receiving desensitizing injections.

IF I HAVE OTHER ALLERGIES, SHOULD I BE TESTED FOR BEE STINGS?

No! Even though you may be more likely to develop a bee allergy than someone who is nonatopic (nonallergic), testing for bee sting allergy should only be done if allergic sensitivity is suspected, i.e., when there is a history of allergic reaction following an actual bee sting. The testing itself may induce sensitivity, or even result in a life-threatening reaction; such tests should not be used to screen individuals simply because they have other allergies.

IF I AM ALLERGIC TO YELLOW JACKETS, CAN I ALSO BE SENSITIVE TO HONEYBEES?

Yes! Stinging insects such as the wasp, yellow jacket, hornet, and the honeybee share common allergenic components. These insects belong to the order *Hymenoptera*. Within this order, the wasp, hornet, and yellow jacket all belong to the Vespid family.

PHYLUM ARTHROPODA

CLASS INSECTA

ORDER HYMENOPTERA

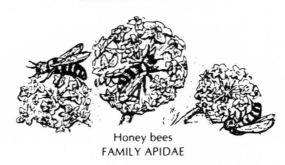

Honey bees
FAMILY APIDAE

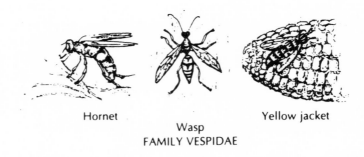

Hornet   Yellow jacket

Wasp
FAMILY VESPIDAE

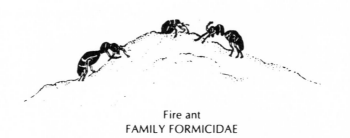

Fire ant
FAMILY FORMICIDAE

Classification of stinging insects.

The honeybee belongs to the Apid family and shares some allergens with the Vespids. If you are allergic to the yellow jacket, you are *most likely* to react to other vespids, but you may also be sensitive to the other members of the honeybee family. For all practical purposes, allergy to bumblebees is essentially the same as allergy to honeybees.

WHAT IS BEE VENOM?

Venom is a complex mixture of various chemicals. The main component of honeybee venom is a protein-like substance called *mellitin*; mellitin causes pain and swelling after a sting. Other components are toxic to nerves. Phospholipase-A, an enzyme, is present in small amounts and is the most important allergenic component.

The venoms of yellow jackets, wasps, and hornets (vespids) contain no mellitin, but do contain similar substances that cause even more intense pain. A principal allergen in vespids is antigen 5. Honeybee venom and the venom of vespids also have components in common.

Bee venom is toxic. A sufficient dose of it can be fatal to a nonallergic individual. It has been estimated that 500 simultaneous stings would be fatal to most.

WHAT ARE KILLER BEES?

Killer bees originate from the mellow European honeybee and the aggressive African honeybee. These African bees make more honey than European and thus were brought to South America for research. Unfortunately, there was an accident and they escaped to the wild. After crossbreeding with the European honeybee, the resultant hybrid became the *Africanized killer bees*. Swarms of these Africanized killer bees have been migrating north through Mexico to Texas, and are now arriving in California. They kill by multiple toxic stings, and not necessarily by allergic reactions. It is really important to avoid risk factors and stay clear of their habitat, which is often a subterranean nest. With ordinary honeybees, it is usually necessary to step on or disturb them in order to provoke a sting. With Africanized killer bees, you shouldn't even risk looking at them cross-eyed!

How Many People Die from Bee Stings?

In 2621 BC, the first fatal reaction from a wasp or hornet sting was recorded in hieroglyphics on the walls of the tomb of the Egyptian King Menes. In the United States about 40 deaths occur each year from such insects as the hornet, wasp, and honeybee. Although allergy to bee stings is more common in younger patients, fatal reactions occur more often in older adults who are more susceptible to the cardiovascular complications of anaphylactic shock. For every death, however, there are thousands of severe and near-fatal reactions.

Who Should Be Given Shots for Bee Sting Allergies?

Immunotherapy should be reserved for those who have a definite history of systemic reaction to a bee sting, with positive results on tests specific for *Hymenoptera* venom. These reactions include difficulty breathing, fainting, and generalized hives. Children whose reaction is limited to hives may not need allergy shots. Progressive local reactions are warning signs of subsequent systemic reactions. Patients should carry a medical emergency kit containing adrenalin and antihistamines.

Researchers are developing criteria to determine how lengthy allergy shot treatments should be for those with bee sting allergy. Some sufferers may actually be *cured* of their allergy, with permanent alleviation being achieved after five years of full dose treatment.

How Can I Avoid Stings?

The key to avoiding stings is understanding the habits of bees and vespids (*see* box on opposite page). Honeybees will not fly when the temperature is less than 55 degrees and will also not fly on cloudy days. They are found around lakes and swimming pools.

Bees are attracted to red objects, so dark or drab colors are recommended. Wear long sleeves and avoid shorts. Walking barefoot is an invitation to trouble; so is wearing perfume. Of course, swatting at bees will provoke a sting.

> **RISK FACTORS FOR BEE STINGS**
> - Truck drivers—open windows
> - Rural outdoor workers—gardeners and farmers
> - Telephone and electrical linemen
> - Beekeepers
> - Floral clothing and perfumes
> - Barefoot in the park and by the pool
> - Late summer cookouts

In most urban communities, the keeping of beehives is illegal. Bees journey for many miles from their hives and wild swarms can settle in trees or around houses. If possible, a beekeeper should remove any hive you may find. Remember, worker bees exposed to insecticide are irritable and are more likely to sting.

Wasps are found around houses, under eaves and behind gutters, while hornets are found in trees and shrubs; their nests may be knocked down and burned. Yellow jackets, like hornets are however found in the ground. They are particularly likely to sting in the fall when the last aggressive, hungry survivors of a colony are attracted to meat and garbage. They are found around picnic areas and around restaurant kitchens. Fast-acting pesticides may be helpful in local control of vespids, but it may be best to consult a professional exterminator.

SHOULD I CARRY AN EMERGENCY KIT?

Positively! Life-threatening edema of the larynx (voice box), wheezing, and anaphylactic shock can occur within minutes of an insect sting. The sensitive person should carry Adrenalin, which can reverse the voice-box swelling and shock. The kits, whether commercial or personally set up, should contain injectable adrenalin and an oral preparation of antihistamines. The use of the adrenalin should be discussed with your physician; the dose will vary with age and weight, and caution should be observed in those suffering hypertension and heart disease.

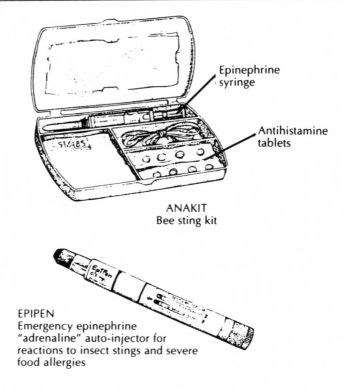

ANAKIT
Bee sting kit

EPIPEN
Emergency epinephrine
"adrenaline" auto-injector for
reactions to insect stings and severe
food allergies

Bee sting kit.

Emergency adrenalin should be used only if systemic symptoms such as respiratory distress, itching, or hives develop. The antihistamine in the kit should be taken after any sting. Antihistamines alone may cause drowsiness, so be careful when driving after taking them.

7

Allergy Shots

How Do Allergy Shots Work?
What Are Allergy Shots?
What Allergens Can Be Used?
When Should I Consider Taking Allergy Shots?
Should I Take Allergy Shots If I Am Pregnant?
Which Diseases Are Helped by Immunotherapy?
How Soon Do Allergy Shots Take Effect?
Do Allergy Shots Always Work?
How Often Must I Take My Allergy Shots?
What Reactions Can I Expect From Allergy Shots?
Is the Dose of Allergy Shots Important?
What Happens If I Stop My Allergy Shots for
  a Few Months?
How Long Will I Have to Take Allergy Shots?
Should Babies Receive Allergy Shots?
May I Take Allergy Shots at Home?
Do Allergy Shots Hurt?
How Expensive Are Allergy Shots?

How Do Allergy Shots Work?

Immunotherapy by means of allergy shots alters your immune system in several ways. First, the shots stimulate your production of the immunoglobulin G (IgG) antibody that is specific for the allergen contained in the allergy extracts. This antibody blocks the normally inhaled allergens from attaching to your sensitized mast cells. Consequently, the mast cells cannot release histamine and other mediators of your allergic response. Additionally, the quantities of secreted gamma globulin (both IgG and IgA) are increased in your nasal passages.

Second, immunotherapy makes your mast cells less responsive to allergenic stimuli. This is like hearing the ticking of a clock while trying to sleep. At first, the tick-tocks may keep you awake, but they become less irritating later as you adapt or become tolerant to the ticking noise. Likewise, the mast cells in your nose, eyes, and lungs become less reactive or more tolerant to the allergenic stimuli.

The third mechanism by which allergy shots work is through the body's production of suppressor lymphocyte cells that turn the immune system off so that it can't manufacture quite so many harmful IgE allergic antibodies. With fewer IgE antibodies available to attach to mast cells, histamine release is inhibited. Hay fever patients usually show an increase in their specific IgE allergy antibody levels at the end of the pollen season; but the opposite happens when an allergy sufferer takes allergy shots—the specific IgE allergic antibody level actually falls at the end of the pollen season.

What Are Allergy Shots?

Allergy shots contain extracts of the substances to which you are allergic. These extracts are made by mixing specific allergens together in a special solution of salt water. Some extracts contain precipitated antigens for delayed absorption into the body tissues; these are useful for highly sensitive allergics.

Allergy extracts have been manufactured since 1911. They have always been helpful for many patients, but there have also

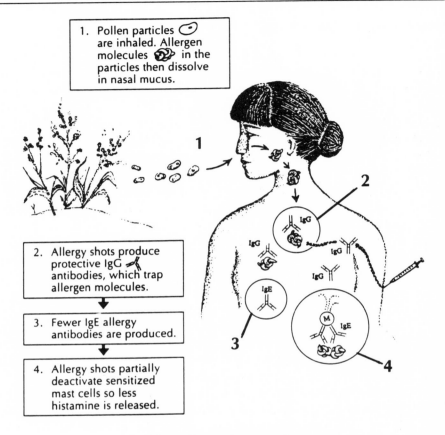

How allergy shots work.

been treatment failures. Many allergics who did not respond to allergy shots in the past were probably not receiving adequate amounts of the specific allergen. For example, dust extracts 20 years ago contained little or no dust mite allergen.

Identification of many specific chemical allergens has now been carried out and has led to the manufacture of new potent and pure allergy extracts for shots—*standardized* extracts. The better the extract, the more successful the results.

Hymenoptera bee sting venoms were the first extracts to be standardized. The newer standardized extracts currently available include those for cat (*Fel d* I), dust mite (*Dermatophagoides pteronyssinus* I and *Dermatophagoides farinae* I), ragweed pollen (antigen E), the important grass pollens, the tree pollens of birch, alder, elder, elm, and oak, and additional weed pollens of Russian thistle, lambs quarter, mugwort, and English plantain. Though these standardized extracts are far more expensive than earlier ones, the results are superior and immunity is more easily achieved with fewer injections.

Allergics often confuse allergy shots with cortisone injections. But cortisone injections are steroids that are often given every year during the pollen season and sometimes all through the year. Steroid side effects can be very harmful and, moreover, can occur even with limited use. Furthermore, a steroid injection does not cure the underlying allergy; in fact, the allergy persists and can even become more severe with continued exposure to such allergy inducers as your cat or ragweed pollen. We, of course, sometimes use cortisone injections for our patients because nothing else provides relief for their most out-of-control symptoms. Though necessary and helpful at times, cortisone shots should not become the mainstay of therapy.

WHAT ALLERGENS CAN BE USED?

Allergy antigen treatment should always include the inhalant allergens to which you are sensitive, but which you cannot easily avoid. Pollens, dust mites, and mold allergens are the most common of these. Bee sting venoms are very effective, and animal danders may be used when you regularly experience significant symptoms after exposure and their avoidance is impossible. Cat allergens are so ubiquitous and cat shots are so effective that we are treating patients with cat antigen far more frequently than in years past. Nevertheless, dander injections are less likely to help when a pet remains in your house continually shedding dander. There is no good evidence that bacterial and food allergy shots are helpful, and food shots may be very dangerous. Incidentally, bakers' asthma is caused by exposure to wheat as an *inhalant*, and not as a food, and allergy shots have been useful in controlling it.

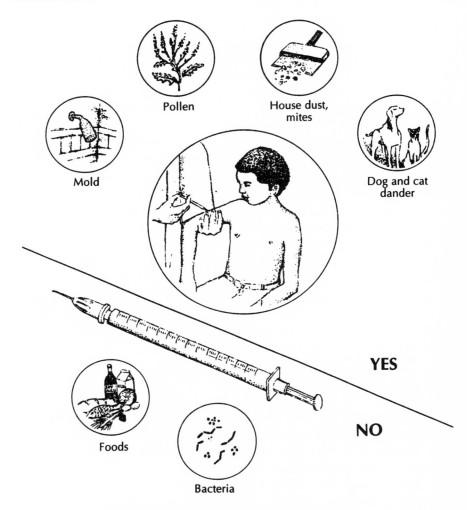

What allergy shots can and cannot do.

WHEN SHOULD I CONSIDER TAKING ALLERGY SHOTS?

Immunotherapy with allergy shots should be considered when your hay fever symptoms are severe enough to interfere with normal daily activities and when medications are not adequate. Significant allergic asthma that correlates with positive skin tests is always an indication that you should take allergy shots.

New medications—steroid sprays and nonsedating antihistamines—are often very effective and many allergics can get through the hay fever season in comfort and do not need allergy shots. For other more sensitive allergics who suffer through the season or who have unavoidable, frequent, serious reactions to cats, dust mites, or molds, medications may not be adequate. Our patients report: "My steroid inhaler used to help, but then stopped—my allergies must be getting worse." or, "That new, nonsedating antihistamine doesn't work as well as it used to. The older antihistamine/decongestants that do work make me too drowsy or jittery or raise my blood pressure. My medicine cabinet looks like a drugstore!" And since the costs of multiple, newly patented medications have skyrocketed, your monthly pharmacy bill is likely to far surpass the cost of allergy shots. Given these circumstances, now may be the time to choose allergy desensitization injections.

Allergy shots are the only treatments that change your basic problem with sensitivity. When the course of therapy is completed, you, as most of our patients, are likely to experience sustained relief.

SHOULD I TAKE ALLERGY SHOTS IF I AM PREGNANT?

Immunotherapy is considered safe for the fetus and desensitization injections are thus generally maintained throughout your pregnancy. Your injections contain the same allergenic material that is absorbed into any mother's body simply by breathing pollen and dust-laden air. Thus every fetus throughout history may be said to have been exposed to airborne allergens. Your allergy shots deliver more of the same naturally occurring substances. As a result, the babies of allergic mothers who had received allergy shots during their pregnancies have been found to develop hay fever less often, and later, than babies from allergic mothers who had not received them. These babies had actually been desensitized during their mother's pregnancy.

To assure the efficacy and safety of allergy shots when you are pregnant, the maintenance dose is usually reduced and the frequency of the injections is increased, which minimizes your risks of adverse systemic reactions—anaphylaxis, in particular, which can cause uterine contractions with obvious consequences. Though anaphylaxis itself can harm your fetus, the allergy shots benefit you at the same time by lessening the need for hay fever and asthma medications. Even so, you should not begin immunotherapy during pregnancy, because the risk of adverse systemic reactions seems to be greatest during the initial period, when the allergen doses are being increased. It is easy enough to wait until after your delivery to start immunotherapy. During pregnancy, you should strive to keep allergy exposures to a minimum.

Incidentally, women of child-bearing age should always let their allergists know when they are considering pregnancy. This will help considerably in planning their treatment programs.

WHICH DISEASES ARE HELPED BY IMMUNOTHERAPY?

The best results are obtained when allergy shots are given for pollen hay fever and asthma. Immunotherapy is also recommended for the control of your nasal and eye symptoms, and for the alleviation of your asthma when it has been caused by dust mites, mold spores, and cat and dog allergens. Your bee sting allergy is best treated with allergy shots, which usually afford excellent curative results.

When eczema is associated with your pollen hay fever, it will sometimes improve with immunotherapy. But often the shots simply make the eczema worse, so that they must then be modified or stopped.

In very limited instances, your hives can be caused by inhalant allergens, which desensitization shots may be helpful in alleviating. Again, hay fever or asthma symptoms are usually associated with hives.

HOW SOON DO ALLERGY SHOTS TAKE EFFECT?

You can expect some improvement from immunotherapy shots after the maintenance dose has been reached. This may take about six months, however, and the degree of improvement is variable, with some allergics soon experiencing good relief and others showing no improvement until a year or two later. But taking your desensitization shots regularly is essential to the effectiveness of the therapy.

Do Allergy Shots Always Work?

Allergy shots are beneficial in 80 to 90% of hay fever cases. Unfortunately, we cannot predict who will respond; some sufferers experience complete relief, whereas others still need to use medications at times. The allergic component of your asthma will also respond in a similar manner. Indeed, allergy shots can successfully relieve your cat or pollen asthma, but the basic tendency to asthma will remain.

Reasons for the failure of immunotherapy shots include your skipping injections, poor control of your environment (cats and dust), failure to achieve an adequately high dose of each of your significant antigens, nonrefrigeration of your extract, and poor quality of the antigen extract used for your shots. The best results are achieved when your properly prescribed antigen extracts are based on the correlation of appropriate skin test results with your clinical symptoms. Your antigen extract formula should be written by an allergist expert in the use of antigens and personally familiar with your condition.

How Often Must I Take My Allergy Shots?

Initially, allergy injections are given once or twice a week, with your dose gradually being increased toward the maintenance dosage. Small starting doses will not provide your long-lasting protection, and adverse reactions are likely to occur if the interval between the increasing doses exceeds one to two weeks. Allergy injections are usually more effective if given to you year-round. Initially, your shots are built up to a dose that is then maintained by injections every two to four weeks. During a subsequent pollen season, the frequency of your shots may again need to be increased. Especially sensitive allergics may require more frequent injections, and weekly injections are sometimes necessary for more than a year.

WHAT REACTIONS CAN I EXPECT FROM ALLERGY SHOTS?

In addition to the benefits you derive from your allergy shots, you may expect some transient reactions since the extract contains substances to which you are specifically allergic. These reactions are usually confined to a small localized area of redness and itching at the site of injection. However, a systemic reaction, involving sneezing, nasal discharge, watery itchy eyes, hives and itching, coughing, and wheezing is always possible. Life-threatening anaphylactic reactions can occur, which explains why you are started with a low dose and then gradually "built up" with each subsequent dose. In this manner you progressively become immune to the antigen so that your body can tolerate the natural exposure. Beta-blockers may increase the risk of reactions. Avoid exercise for two hours after shots.

IS THE DOSE OF ALLERGY SHOTS IMPORTANT?

Yes. Sufferers respond best to allergy shots when they receive the largest dose they can tolerate. Reaching the maximum requires an individualized program from your allergist. Although allergy immunotherapy has been used safely and effectively for years, recent research has been able to determine scientifically the dose necessary for immune response in most patients.

The strength of the antigen is most commonly expressed as the ratio of the weight of the pollen to the weight of water in which it is extracted. Pollen extracts are most commonly manufactured as 1:20 concentrates. Immunotherapy may begin with a concentration of 1:200,000 or 1:2,000,000. The eventual maintenance dose should ideally be 1:200 or greater. Strengths are sometimes expressed as a concentration of protein, and in this system the maintenance dosage will be given from bottles labeled, for example, 10,000 protein/nitrogen units per milliliter (cc); the higher the number the more antigen in each vial.

The new *standardized* and highly effective allergy extracts come in concentrations expressed as Allergy Units or Biological Allergy Units. With these freshly standardized measurements, the optimal dose ranges from 1000 to 4000 Allergy Units per allergen per injection. This high dose regimen needs to be individualized for each patient and monitored by your allergist. For clinical improvement, you should achieve your highest tolerated dose up to this optimal recommended dose. Sensitive patients can achieve improvement at lower doses.

WHAT HAPPENS IF I STOP MY ALLERGY SHOTS FOR A FEW MONTHS?

If a long absence is necessary because of work or a vacation, your dose is first reduced, and then built back up at weekly intervals. The amount of the reduction depends on your sensitivity and the history of your prior systemic reactions, if any, on the previous maintenance dose, on the length of time you have been on immunotherapy, and on the time since your last shot. In your year-round maintenance program, a vacation should pose no problems. After two or three weeks, little or no adjustment of a top maintenance dose should be necessary. If three or four months are missed, you will certainly need a dosage reduction and a buildup period of weekly treatments. We regularly prepare extracts that our patients can take on extended vacations. These can be administered by a local physician, aboard cruise ships by the ship's physician, or in the Emergency Department of a hospital. You should check to make sure that these physicians have some familiarity with allergy antigen injections and that they have on hand the medications needed to treat any systemic reaction that occurs.

HOW LONG WILL I HAVE TO TAKE ALLERGY SHOTS?

Treatment should last a minimum of four to five years to give you the best chance for long-standing benefit. Generally, children are more able to discontinue immunotherapy after this length of time. On the other hand, many adults must continue with allergy shots for a longer period.

If you wait to stop treatment until after two symptom-free years have passed, your symptoms will be less likely to recur. In the case of bee sting venom immunotherapy, a top dose of 100 micrograms per injection per month for five years may confer permanent protection after shots are stopped. Skin testing must be repeated to demonstrate a reversal of sensitivity.

Should Babies Receive Allergy Shots?

It is extremely unusual for an infant to develop allergy symptoms to multiple pollens during the first year or two of life. There has not really been much time for repeated exposure and increased sensitization, especially for seasonal pollens. However, we do see infant allergy to house dust mites, molds, and animal danders in this age group.

Skin testing can be done (and can be positive) at any age; however, the number of antigens for testing is much smaller during the first year or two, and not as many skin tests are necessary.

Allergy in the first two years of life is often related to foods, and asthma is usually triggered by viruses. The treatment is elimination of the food in question and avoidance of crowded conditions—not allergy shots.

May I Take Allergy Shots at Home?

Allergy injections contain a selection of antigens to which you are allergic. Each injection carries a risk of anaphylaxis and shock. The treatment schedule planned by your allergist should be individualized to minimize this risk. According to the National Institutes of Health, as well as a position paper from the American Academy of Allergy and Immunology, the patient should be observed for 20 to 30 minutes after allergy shots. The observer should have readily available the equipment and drugs necessary to treat shock and respiratory failure.

Getting injections at home is risky business. However, if you receive them in your physician's office, a serious reaction can be treated immediately. In rural areas where there is no physician, the benefits of immunotherapy may necessitate home injections. But with rare exceptions, the treatment should be given in your physician's office.

Do Allergy Shots Hurt?

Maybe a little. Injections are given with the smallest needles. Usually, 1 cc or milliliter—only 16 drops—of antigen or less is injected just under the skin. Itching and swelling may result, but discomfort from the injection itself is minimal. Even young children do not cry once they get over the fear of the initial injections.

How Expensive Are Allergy Shots?

Allergy shots range from $15.00 to $25.00 in the West and up to $35.00 in the metropolitan East. This is the price for every allergy shot treatment, whether your extract is divided into two or three shots or is given all in the same injection. Your cost during the first year could be anywhere from $800.00 to $1800.00. Thereafter, as the interval between injections increases, your cost should decrease. The antigen extract used for your injection may be billed separately from the injections themselves, and this may cost from $150.00 to $300.00 per year. Remember that in time the cost of allergy injections will be offset by your savings in allergy and asthma medications.

The new venom extract for bee sting allergy is very expensive and the costs become much higher. This is reflected in the special charge for venom skin testing as well.

While you receive immunotherapy, your reactions are closely observed; your progress is monitored and necessary modifications of your dose and extract are made by trained nurses and your allergy specialist. The treatment visit includes careful record-keeping and occasional prescription refills. Take the time to ask these professionals any questions you may have regarding your allergies.

Of course, with most HMOs and PPOs the reimbursement is predetermined and you are usually only responsible for a copayment. Allergy patients should carefully choose an insurance company that covers allergy care.

8

Drug Allergies

WHICH ARE THE MOST ALLERGENIC DRUGS?

Any drug may cause an allergic reaction, but penicillin is the most common cause of drug allergy. It has been widely studied, and skin testing can be done in order to confirm or rule out penicillin sensitivity. If you are truly allergic to penicillin, then you should also avoid ampicillin, amoxicillin, and the other penicillin-related antibiotics (cloxacillin, etc.). Cephalosporins (Keflex, Ceclor, Ceftin) are also related to penicillin and may possibly evoke an allergic response. If you have an allergic reaction to one antibiotic, you are at considerably increased risk for allergic sensitivity to other antibiotics whether they are chemically related or not.

Sulfa (sulfonamide) allergy can cause severe hives, and may occasionally cause a life-threatening reaction called *erythema multiforme*. This antibiotic (Gantrisin, Gantanol) is widely used for urinary tract (bladder) infections. Currently, sulfa is often prescribed by pediatricians in combination with another antibiotic (the combination is called Pediazole) for middle ear infections because bacterial resistance to ampicillin and amoxicillin has rendered them ineffective. For similar reasons, Septra/Bactrim (a combination of sulfa and trimethoprim) is used for respiratory, bladder, and sinus infections. This drug is also used in AIDS patients for a life-threatening pneumonia, Pneumocystis, and they frequently become sensitized to Septra/Bactrim. Certain diuretics (thiazides; Lasix) are sulfonamides and may cause allergic reactions in some patients with sulfa allergy.

Tetracycline and erythromycin are frequently used broad-spectrum antibiotics. They have a much lower incidence of allergic potential; nevertheless, a patient may become sensitized. Beware of sun exposure if you are taking tetracycline derivatives.

For all these and other reasons, antibiotics should not be taken indiscriminately by people with allergies. The best treatment for drug allergy is simple avoidance. Luckily for those with drug allergies, new classes of antibiotics are constantly being developed, for example, quinolones (Cipro and others), and these offer promise of effective replacement of the known allergy-inducing drugs in the management of infections.

Seizure medications (Dilantin, phenobarbital, and Tegretol) are also known to have caused prolonged allergic skin rashes and should always be considered possible causes of suspicious new skin outbreaks. There is a very low incidence of allergy to human insulin; if local hives appear at the injection site, a switch from NPH to Regular or Lente is usually all that is necessary since this reaction is probably to the protamine in NPH. The new synthetic human insulin is an exact copy of your insulin and should not cause the sort of significant allergic reactions that the still widely used beef and pork insulins have more commonly produced.

How Do Drugs Cause Allergy?

After you take a drug, it breaks down into substances known as haptens that can cause allergy. These haptens combine with proteins in your body, thereby producing an allergic sensitization. In this manner, your body may produce the allergic antibody IgE after a drug is taken. When the same drug is subsequently taken again, the pre-formed antibody combines with the drug's hapten and your allergy reaction occurs. Anaphylaxis, whether mild or severe, can result from such drug allergies, and the spectrum of reaction ranges from mild itching to shock and death.

Other reactive antibodies that cause such symptoms as easy bruising, hemorrhage, and anemia by destroying red blood cells may also be formed. When the drug combines with the antibody, the resulting complex can deposit in your tissues, causing manifestations in the kidneys. Fortunately, this reaction is not common. Lymphocytes (a white blood cell type of your immune system) may themselves become sensitized to drugs, causing skin rashes.

The altered metabolism in AIDS patients is what often leads to a high incidence of drug allergy—especially to sulfa. And finally, some drugs cause reactions by releasing histamine from mast cells, for example, X-ray dyes and codeine.

Some Common Drugs and Their Nonallergic Side Effects		
Drug	Effect	Side effects
Dilantin (diphenylhydantoin)	Prevents seizures	Overgrowth of gums
Aspirin and other NSAIDs (ibuprofen, naprosyn)	Relieves pain	Minute bleeding spots in the intestines, asthma
Erythromycin	Kills bacteria	Nausea and stomachache
Antacids	Relieves pain of heartburn	Constipation or diarrhea
Birth control pills	Prevents ovulation	Increased incidence of stroke
Theophylline	Relieves wheezing	Irritability, stomachache, and headache
Chlorpheniramine	Dries allergic secretions	Drowsiness
Capoten, Vasotec	Lowers blood pressure	Cough, severe swelling
Calcium channel blockers (Calan, Procardia)	Lowers blood pressure	Swollen ankles

WHAT ARE THE SIDE EFFECTS OF DRUGS?

Many drugs have more effects than the one you take them for (*see* box). In the case of antihistamines, relief from itching may be the desired effect, whereas drowsiness is a common side effect. Frequently, patients confuse side effects with allergies. It is important to distinguish between true allergy and side effects. If you have experienced an allergic reaction to a medication, you must thereafter avoid that drug because a second exposure may lead to a more serious reaction. On the other hand, the potential benefit of a drug may be so great that you are willing to endure some side effects.

CAN ASPIRIN CAUSE ALLERGIES?

Acetylsalicylic acid, commonly known as aspirin, can severely exacerbate asthma, especially if you have nasal polyps and chronic sinusitis. The asthma typically occurs 20 minutes after you take the aspirin and the attack is intractable and sometimes fatal. Aspirin can also trigger hives and swelling of the larynx. Aspirin intolerance is present in at least 5% of asthmatics and in 1% of the general population.

An accurate history of your aspirin intake accompanied by exacerbation of symptoms within 30 minutes is sufficient proof that aspirin intolerance exists. Clues to the presence of aspirin sensitivity include a persistent, watery, nasal discharge and nasal polyps. Marked improvement of your symptoms after aspirin elimination is also sufficient proof.

If you have aspirin intolerance, all aspirin-containing products must be avoided. Read labels! Many over-the-counter pain and cold preparations such as Alka-Seltzer and Coricidin contain aspirin. Anti-inflammatory pain-relieving medications, which are commonly used to treat arthritis and bursitis, also aggravate intolerance in aspirin-sensitive patients. Some of these nonsteroidal anti-inflammatory drugs (NSAIDs) are indomethacin (Indocin), phenylbutazone (Butazolidin), ibuprofen (Motrin, Advil, etc.), tolmetin (Tolectin), piroxicam (Feldene), naproxen (Naprosyn), diclofenac (Voltaren), ketorolac (Toradol), and other preparations that belong to the same rapidly expanding family of drugs.

Aspirin-sensitive allergics have reportedly experienced difficulty after ingesting tartrazine yellow food coloring (FD&C No. 5). We have not seen this, however, in our practices. Tartrazine is found in many foods, particularly orange-flavored drinks, and is used to make some foods appear rich in eggs or butter. Oranges have even been injected with tartrazine for better color. Elimination and challenge testing with tartrazine may be indicated and should only be done under the supervision of your allergist.

Fortunately, most aspirin-intolerant patients can tolerate acetaminophen (Tylenol, Panadol, Liquiprin), which is useful for reducing fever and treating pain, though it still will not reduce the inflammation of arthritis or bursitis. However, the nonsteroidal anti-inflammatory drug salsalate (Disalcid) may be tolerated in patients with aspirin sensitivity.

CAN I HAVE A SECOND REACTION TO X-RAY DYES?

If you have had an anaphylactic-like reaction with itching, difficulty breathing, or shock when you took the radiocontrast dyes used for such X-ray procedures as IVPs, CT scans, and angiograms, this reaction can happen again, and may prove even more severe and life-threatening. Your physician can premedicate you before your next X-ray with a radiocontrast dye by using prednisone and antihistamines. With these medications, the risk of a repeat reaction can be significantly reduced. The reaction occurs because the dye releases histamine from your cells. New (and far more expensive) low osmolality dyes can be substituted, and these greatly reduce the incidence of allergics reactions. There is no relationship between the allergic-like reactions caused by radiocontrast dyes and those of seafood allergy. Your allergy to fish and shellfish is the result of allergy antibodies directed at specific fish proteins and not to the direct response of your cells to iodine.

CAN SKIN TESTS BE USED TO DETECT DRUG ALLERGY?

Penicillin and some cephalosporins (Ceclor and Ceftin) give reliable skin test results. Testing for other antibiotics (sulfa) is under development. Special test materials are necessary, and commercially available reagents as well as those prepared by your allergist may be used.

Skin testing may also be helpful in the preliminary evaluation of allergy to local anesthetics such as Xylocaine. If your skin tests are at first negative, increasing doses are given sequentially and you will be observed for untoward reactions. Fortunately, allergic reactions to local anesthetics are rare. In the past Novocain caused some allergic reactions—for the dentist (a dermatitis) as well as the patient. Xylocaine and Carbocaine have replaced Novocain and there are some other newer local anesthetics as well. You should see an allergist if you have a history of an adverse reaction to local anesthetics. We have seen many patients who have declined local anesthetics and thus needlessly endured painful procedures because they erroneously believed they were allergic to local anesthetics.

Here is one such case. We were asked to see a patient referred from the hospital Emergency Room. She had been injected with Xylocaine in preparation for suturing a deep shaving laceration on her leg, and within minutes had developed full-blown anaphylactic shock. Fortunately, she could be given immediate care in our hospital. Further history taking revealed that she had been developing progressively severe episodes of hives and swelling that seemed to be associated with her menses. She reported that she was not taking any medications. Skin testing and subsequent titration challenge testing to Xylocaine gave entirely negative results, indicating that Xylocaine was not the problem. Upon repeated questioning she recalled that she had been taking Motrin for menstrual cramps for at least the last six months. Almost by habit she had reached into the medicine cabinet to take a Motrin the morning she had shaved since this was the first day of her period. She lived within blocks of the Emergency Room so the Xylocaine had been injected at about the time that her reaction to Motrin started. Skin tests ruled out one suspect, Xylocaine, while the historical evidence convicted the other—Motrin. Her monthly episodes of hives and swelling did not recur after the Motrin was discontinued.

WHO SHOULD BE TESTED FOR DRUG ALLERGIES?

This is a thorny problem. For each allergic person, the approach must be individualized. If you have a vague, unclear history of allergy to penicillin and its derivatives, or to some cephalosporin, and the use of antibiotic is necessary to treat your recurrent infections, then skin testing is indicated. If your skin tests are positive, then you are allergic and you must avoid penicillin. Negative skin tests are not completely reliable and may miss up to 5% of those who are truly allergic. A subsequent oral challenge may be administered by your allergist to confirm that you are, in fact, able to tolerate the antibiotic.

A six-year-old child with recurrent middle ear infections has come to our office with a history of a rash while taking amoxicillin for a febrile illness. His pediatrician wants to know whether penicillins can be prescribed again in the future. The child's skin testing results are negative and the oral challenge is also negative. Our conclusion is that the child can tolerate penicillin now, and that penicillin can be prescribed in the future. The rash, we assume, was caused by a viral infection.

If a clear history indicates a high probability of an allergic drug reaction, then you may take the following measures. Allergy skin testing is carried out only when a specific antibiotic therapy is both imminent and necessary, and there is no good reasonable alternative drug. Testing for the possible future use of penicillins when there is a clear history of drug allergy is not advised. If 10 years or so have passed since the probable reaction, there is a 90% chance that you have lost your sensitivity, and that testing or challenge without any imminent need for therapy may only serve to resensitize you unnecessarily for another 10 years.

A 45-year-old man came for evaluation of drug allergy. He had a definite history of an allergic reaction to penicillin 15 years earlier. His ear, nose, and throat specialist wanted him to be tested for penicillin to be used in possible future sinusitis treatment. We told him that he could be tested only when he might actually need a penicillin drug if there were no good alternative antibiotics. We suggested that with his next infection he should first use a cephalosporin and continue to avoid penicillins. Though cephalosporins are related to penicillins, the incidence of allergy for cephalosporins in penicillin-allergic patients is the same as that for antibiotics not related to penicillin.

Sometimes there is a positive history of allergy to penicillin and a positive skin test, but it is nonetheless necessary. A patient with lupus and a history of penicillin allergy was admitted to the hospital for Listeria meningitis and needed amoxicillin. No other drug could be used. Fortunately, skin testing was negative so that she could receive an intravenous test dose and thereafter continue with treatment. If the skin tests were positive, oral or intravenous desensitization might have been done.

There is also a blood test for penicillin allergy. This has limited use in penicillin allergy screening, but if the test gives a positive result, you are surely allergic and should not take penicillin. If the test results are negative, further allergy consultation is necessary. Still other, new tests are currently under development.

Aspirin allergy is a troublesome problem for many patients. If aspirin causes your asthma, it is often obvious; however, some patients may only manifest changes when special spirometry testing of the patient's breathing is carried out following sequential, incremental, small doses of aspirin—with spirometry evaluation 20 minutes after each dose. This is a specialized test and should be done only under careful medical supervision. Other nonsteroidal anti-inflammatory drugs such as Motrin and Naprosyn should be strictly avoided if there is any sensitivity.

If aspirin causes your hives, you may sometimes be able to tolerate other anti-inflammatory drugs. This is very important for those with arthritis. Serial testing with small doses of a selected alternative drug may allow you to identify a nonsteroidal anti-inflammatory drug you can tolerate. This is true even if you are sensitive to another nonsteroidal anti-inflammatory drug. For example, if you are allergic to aspirin you might wish to be tested for Motrin, or if you are sensitive to Naprosyn, then tested for Feldene. The testing must be followed by appropriate periods of observation for each increasing dose.

WHAT ABOUT ANTIBIOTIC CREAMS?

An allergic skin rash caused by the antibiotic neomycin in Neosporin cream can be a problem, but not as common as once thought. The neomycin component can cause a contact dermatitis similar to that of poison oak. Bacitracin and Polysporin (OTC) and Bactroban (Rx only) do not contain neomycin.

If you have a diffuse skin infection, then a penicillin derivative or oral erythromycin may be necessary. Bactroban is effective for impetigo and infected eczema.

SHOULD I TAKE PENICILLIN IF I AM ALLERGIC TO IT? WHAT IF I REALLY NEED IT?

Yes, you can be desensitized so that penicillin treatment is feasible when absolutely necessary. For severe life-threatening infections of the heart, and in other rare circumstances, penicillin is the only effective drug and thus must be used. If there is severe penicillin allergy and no other drug can be used, a special "rush program" of desensitization can be carried out in a hospital intensive care unit. Multiple doses of penicillin are administered minutes apart until the strength needed for treatment is achieved without adverse side effects.

CAN DENTAL DISCLOSING TABLETS CAUSE ALLERGY?

Disclosing tablets contain a staining dye and are used to show plaque on teeth. Several kinds of disclosing tablets (Xpose, Red Cote) also contain the antibiotic erythromycin, a potent photosensitizing drug when it is applied topically. When the tablet is dissolving in your mouth, the solution may come into contact with the lips. If you fail to wash the solution off, subsequent exposure to sunlight may result in a serious photoallergic reaction: swelling, blistering, and crusting of your lips.

CAN I BECOME ALLERGIC TO MY ALLERGY MEDICATIONS?

Fortunately, allergy and asthma medications rarely cause drug allergies. Antihistamines such as diphenhydramine may cause allergy when they are used on the skin. Reactions to antihistamines in eyedrops are possible, but rarely occur.

Some over-the-counter allergy medications contain aspirin, which frequently can cause allergy and allergy-like reactions. Allergy and asthma drugs may also contain coal-tar dyes such as tartrazine, which is thought to cause problems, though rarely. There are reported incidences of allergy to cortisone, and specifically with Medrol. You can also develop an allergic contact dermatitis to the preservative in cortisone creams, though the ointments usually have no preservatives. Excessive use of prescription-strength topical cortisones can cause a rash that can be confused with allergy—the rash clears when you stop the cream or ointment.

DOES CODEINE CAUSE ALLERGIES?

When codeine is injected into normal skin, histamine is released from the mast cells in the skin and an itchy wheal and flare (hives) results. Some people are particularly sensitive to the action of this drug and experience generalized hives and itching when they take codeine by mouth. No allergy antibody is involved; however, this reaction is a serious *side effect* that may become progressively more severe. Codeine can also cause a true allergy reaction, but this is less frequent. Related drugs to be avoided include such natural and synthetic narcotics as morphine, Demerol, and Talwin.

CAN ONE DEVELOP A COCAINE ALLERGY?

Inhaling cocaine into the nose ("snorting") may result in typical allergy-like symptoms: clear nasal discharge and conjunctival irritation with watery, itchy eyes. This is a common side effect of the drug, and prolonged use may result in destruction of the nasal septum. Rare instances of true allergic reactions (anaphylaxis and asthma) have been reported. A sane person would not even try cocaine or crack.

DOES THE SUN CAUSE DRUG REACTIONS?

Yes. Some drugs, such as sulfa, tranquilizers (Thorazine), and a few infrequently prescribed forms of tetracycline can render your skin exquisitely sensitive to the sun; even short exposure can then result in severe sunburns.

In the presence of sunlight, these photosensitizing drugs combine with proteins in your skin to form allergenic complexes. When you take the drug a second or third time and then go out in the sun, a severe allergic skin rash can develop. Antiseptic agents (such as the halogenated salicylamides used in soaps) may cause this reaction; sulfa drugs and thiazides (which are used for diuretic blood pressure control) may also be associated with this reaction. If you cannot avoid a drug to which you are photosensitive, you must avoid the sun, or use sunscreens with UVA and UVB protection having an SPF #15. The common sunscreen PABA and other newer sunscreen chemicals can cause skin allergies, but alternatives are available. Micropulverized titanium dioxide blocks the rays of the sun without penetrating or interacting with the skin, like an invisible zinc oxide—remember the white nose of your lifeguard.

CAN I HAVE MULTIPLE DRUG ALLERGIES?

Yes. Some people have a tendency to develop drug allergy because of the way they metabolize medications. If your body breaks down penicillin and if the breakdown products combine with certain proteins, then you may be such an individual with a potential for drug allergy. The development of one allergy sends up a red flag that you are at risk for developing sensitivity to other potentially allergenic drugs. Twenty percent of patients with a penicillin allergy can become allergic to erythromycin, a completely unrelated drug. Clearly medications should only be taken when necessary, especially if you have experienced a drug allergy.

CAN I PREVENT DRUG ALLERGIES?

You certainly can! Don't take antibiotics every time you might just have a viral infection such as the flu. "Shotgun" treatment may unnecessarily sensitize you to drugs that you may later need for a specific severe illness.

Good nutrition (chicken soup!) and rest are necessary for your immune system to fight infections effectively. But remember, of course, that antibiotics are required for many bacterial infections, and can be safely prescribed if your doctor knows your specific allergies.

WHAT IS G-6-PD?

G-6-PD, glucose-6-phosphate-dehydrogenase, is an enzyme necessary to maintain the integrity of red blood cells; that is, to keep them from leaking oxygen-carrying hemoglobin. A partial deficiency of this enzyme is an inherited condition that most frequently affects black males. When G-6-PD-deficient people take certain drugs, such as Primaquine (for malaria), sulfa, and phenacetin (in APCs, aspirin, phenacetin, caffeine; Empirin), their red blood cells break up and anemia results. Interestingly, eating fava beans can cause anemia, called *favism*, in those affected. This drug-caused anemia is nonallergic and is thus considered an idiosyncratic response.

WHAT IS ERYTHEMA MULTIFORME?

Erythema multiforme is a skin rash manifested during a severe life-threatening reaction called toxic epidermal necrolysis (TEN). The skin lesions are large and have a "target" appearance: circular, red, and raised with a clear area in the middle. The reaction can dangerously include the mucous membranes, resulting in blisters of the mouth, eyes, and genitals, with scarring of these membranes. This manifestation is called Stevens-Johnson syndrome. Despite intensive medical intervention, this reaction can be fatal. Severe hives are sometimes incorrectly called erythema multiforme; but hives of any severity do not have the implications of TEN.

Erythema multiforme most frequently results from an allergic reaction to sulfa, although other antibiotics and medications have been implicated. Drugs to avoid if you are allergic to sulfa (sulforamide), include: TMS (trimethoprim sulfa, Septra, Bactrim), sulfisoxazole (Gantrisin), sulfamethoxazole (Gantanol), and sulfisoxazole (erythromycin, Pediazole). The common diuretic "water pill," Dyazide contains hydrochlorothiazide and triamterene; and the thiazide diuretics cross-react with sulfa sensitivity, and should also be avoided. Since many drugs contain sulfa, you must, if you have sulfa allergies, always check with your physician and your pharmacist to make sure that you are not given a drug that may prove harmful.

Allergics with sulfa sensitivity, when reading the ingredients of their asthma tablets, solutions, and syrups, see that they contain albuterol sulfate and then occasionally panic. Sulfates of any sort are salts of the element sulfur and thus are not related to sulfa drugs. Likewise, patients who wheeze when exposed to sulfites need not be concerned about "sulfates" on many medica-

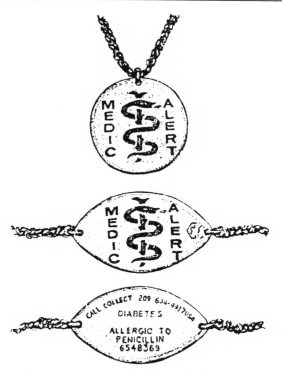

Medic Alert necklace (top) and both sides of Medic Alert bracelet.

tion labels. Don't be inappropriately concerned—*but always ask questions*. Better to be safe than sorry.

Should I Wear a Medic Alert Bracelet or Necklace?

Some people should. A Medic Alert* necklace looks like a dog tag, and provides information about your medical condition and allergies in case of an emergency.

You should wear one if you have experienced a life-threatening reaction either to a drug such as penicillin, to a bee sting, or to a particular food such as peanuts. Severe asthmatics, particularly children, should also wear one.

*Medic Alert is a nonprofit organization: 2323 Colorado Avenue, Turlock, California 95380.

9

New and Controversial Issues— Behavioral and Body Systems

9 New and Controversial Issues

Should I Get a Room Ionizer?
Will Meditation Help My Allergy?
Do I Have to Sit Still to Meditate?
Should I Seek Acupuncture Treatment?
What Are Urine Shots?

WHAT IS ANECDOTAL EVIDENCE?

As physicians treating patients, we make many observations regarding our patients' diseases and their responses to various therapies. Along with the knowledge we acquired in medical school and in our subsequent specialty training, this accumulated learning greatly enhances our "clinical experience." It is this steadily increasing clinical experience that transforms the student of medical texts into a physician. As we gain more experience, we become better equipped to search for more effective methods of diagnosis and treatment. Often great advances have come from the observation or treatment of a single patient. In the 1800s, Edward Jenner observed that milkmaids who had been infected with cowpox were spared the ravages of smallpox. He had the courage to perform the first vaccination—purposely injecting a young boy with a mild disease (cowpox) in order to protect him from smallpox. Over the last century, immunization against smallpox became a universal health measure, and is so successful that the World Health Organization has recently determined smallpox to have been eliminated as a threat to human health.

On the other hand, isolated observations may bear no relationship to the truth. We teach this to our children—saying that feeling a bump on your head does not necessarily mean that the sky is falling. Thus patient testimonies do not prove that a medical treatment is effective, or even safe. In medicine, we refer to the use of such testimony to prove the worth of a new treatment as *anecdotal evidence*; it is always interesting, perhaps helpful, but not necessarily proof that the therapy works or fails. Consider the case of thymus irradiation, a "cure" for noisy breathing in babies that was popular during the 1940s because of favorable patient testimony and a mistaken perception of efficacy by physicians. This therapy was not only ineffective, but sometimes caused cancer of the thyroid.

New diagnostic methods and treatments must today be subjected to a complete range of scientific studies before they are prescribed by physicians or used by the patient–consumer. Today, Doctor Jenner would need to follow the scientific and ethical standards of Jonas Salk and Albert Sabin in their development of polio vaccines. These are also major considerations in the search for a safe and effective AIDS vaccine.

WHAT IS THE PLACEBO EFFECT?

A placebo is an inactive substance, drug, or treatment given to patients under the guise of being a genuine treatment. Paradoxically, a beneficial clinical response often follows. This is known as the "placebo effect."

The placebo effect is well documented in medicine. Placebo medications can provide some symptomatic relief about 30% of the time. Patients' expectations and faith in therapy explain the effect. The mechanism may be the release of chemicals (endorphins) from the brain that alter perception. The placebo effect is so strong that even clinical investigators have been fooled. If sugar pills are sold as aspirin, the placebo effect is likely to result in more than 30% of patients reporting relief from their pain.

DO SOME *INDIVIDUAL* DOCTORS HAVE SPECIAL KNOWLEDGE ABOUT ALLERGY?

There is no magic in medicine. You should be skeptical of any doctor who claims to have unique, revolutionary, and special methods of diagnosis or treatment. We occasionally hear of a doctor who is the only person in the community who has mastered a new and often dramatic system for healing. Some of these "cures" amount to the snake oil of today's therapies and are often uniquely expensive.

The Hippocratic oath requires that physicians teach their skills to others. Valid and proven advances in therapy are readily and rapidly accepted, and soon widely adopted. Some examples of this rapid acceptance are the treatment of diabetes mellitus with insulin and the current use of bee venoms for the treatment of bee allergy. Although some procedures, such as the recent gene therapy for the immune disorder, adenosine deaminase deficiency (ADA) must be carried out in special centers (for example, at the University of California at San Francisco and at UCLA), physicians almost universally share their expertise and knowledge with the public and the medical community at large.

They are generally eager to disclose their procedures and encourage medical and scientific scrutiny. When they show any effectiveness, they don't keep their novel therapies to themselves.

ARE THERE DIFFERENT FORMS OF SKIN TESTING?

The most widely used and accepted form of skin testing is the scratch technique that uses concentrates of different allergen extracts. This may be followed by selected intradermal tests that utilize a weaker dilution. Treatment is based on positive tests that have significance in terms of your clinical history. Allergy shots are started at a weak dilution and then slowly progress to stronger dilutions as each dose is tolerated.

There are other techniques that utilize varying dilutions of the same allergens, given in multiple intradermal injections, to determine sensitivity as well as the starting dose for allergy shots; future adjustments of the dose are necessary as they continue. We do not use this alternative technique because high optimal dose therapy has been clearly demonstrated to be most efficacious.

WHAT IS SUBLINGUAL TESTING?

Sublingual testing is an attempt to diagnose allergies by provoking allergy symptoms. The method involves placing drops of diluted allergenic material under the tongue. A positive test is reported when the patient states that symptoms have developed or when the observer notes difficulty in breathing, random eye movements, or lethargy. This method is unreliable and has not yet been tested by objective and reproducible means, such as pulmonary function tests or measurements of nasal swelling through airway flow rates. By contrast, skin tests provoke a measurable reaction in the skin whose correlation to allergy has been proven.

WHAT IS THE NEUTRALIZATION DOSE?

Some practitioners claim that allergic symptoms can be turned off or "neutralized" by administering a dilute concentration of the allergen. This dose is injected or placed as a drop under your tongue (sublingual).

The idea is appealing, but no controlled studies have shown it to be effective. In fact, recent studies have shown the opposite to be true. The best relief with immunotherapy occurs when you receive allergy shots with progressively larger injections of anti-gen—the higher the maintenance dose the greater your relief.

What Is Holistic Medicine and How Does It Relate to Allergy?

"Holistic" comes from the Greek word *holos*, which means whole. Simply, holistic medicine refers to the whole patient; the psyche (mind) and body are one, an inseparable whole. In the extreme, holistic medicine teaches that if we lived in harmony in a pollution-free environment, we would be free of disease—in short, that we now choose our own illnesses.

In the sense of "whole," good allergists are holistic practitioners. They realize that bad habits such as cigaret smoking and poor nutrition contribute to disease. They know that anxiety and unresolved stressful situations in our lives can exacerbate sinusitis as well as asthma. Thus an allergist can help identify the high-risk asthmatic adolescent who is trying to punish a parent by making his or her asthma worse through either treatment noncompliance or negative behavior. Additionally, asthma and allergy specialists are quite aware that air pollution worsens breathing and is detrimental to the health of infants.

A good allergist will help you understand your illness so that you can better live with your allergies, and will teach you how to alter your environment for better health.

Human beings can and will adapt to modern technology and its consequences; the world population today cannot survive without it. The reality is that, though some individuals may become ill from agricultural harmful pesticides, millions may starve without these chemicals. We cannot return to the past. Further, we need to strive to develop nonharmful technology to feed and heal the world—in the Hebrew—*tikkun olam*.

WHAT IS CEREBRAL ALLERGY?

Cerebral allergy is an *alleged* condition in which an individual shows a psychological reaction to environmental substances that are tolerated by nonallergic people. Complaints of difficulty in thinking or moving are wrongly ascribed to an allergic reaction in your brain. There is no evidence that such allergic reactions occur in brain tissue, but changes in blood vessels—spasm or dilatation—are known to contribute to headache symptoms. So far, the evidence for cerebral or brain *allergy* is entirely anecdotal, and further research is necessary before this diagnosis can be made. Some symptoms are actually phobias, a misunderstanding that is being reinforced by some popular magazines and books.

Allergy and asthma can affect your mood. Hay fever is called "fever" because its associated phenomena not limited to the nose, eyes, and lungs, but generalized, include such symptoms as malaise, fatigue, and headache. Though endorphins and neurotransmitters may be involved, there is no evidence for an allergic reaction in the brain.

WHAT IS THE "SICK BUILDING SYNDROME"?

Have you ever been in a building where you can't open the windows? Bacteria and molds may contaminate the air conditioning system. The cooling system uses water storage tanks that cannot be sterilized and a "humidifier syndrome" may develop in exposed patients. Legionnaire's disease, first discovered in a hotel in Philadelphia, is a classic sick-building-syndrome form of pneumonia with flu-like symptoms.

The sick building syndrome more commonly occurs in new office buildings that are sealed, utilizing recirculated air. In addition to bacteria and molds, there may be irritating odors that cause irritation to your skin, throat, eyes, and bronchial tubes, and also cause headaches. These odors may originate from carpeting, furniture, building materials, some paper office supplies, and even copy machines. The offending chemicals may also be "silent" and odorless.

A patient recently came to see us with disorientation and headaches. She worked in the Pathology Department of a hospital and no one believed her until one of the physician pathologists was also affected. It turned out that exhaust fumes from the ambulances were feeding through the ventilation right into the departmental offices, causing their illness.

Standards for air circulation in the workplace may vary, but if you are affected you should know that an air exchange of approximately 20 cubic feet per minute per person should be adequate. The solution lies in adequate ventilation with fresh, clean air.

IS THE CHRONIC FATIGUE SYNDROME CAUSED BY ALLERGY?

This syndrome may or may not exist as a specific unified illness, but it certainly is overdiagnosed. Patients often become obsessively focused on their complaints and inappropriately alter their lives. This is a syndrome with multiple, diffuse components. The main characteristic is a profound, debilitating, and crippling fatigue. The major diagnostic criterion based on your history is the recent development of a fatigue that limits your daily activity to one-half of the previous level. Many minor diagnostic criteria exist. They include symptoms of mild fever, sore throat, muscle aches, headaches, and sleep disturbance. Lymph node enlargement and tenderness is an objective, measurable finding.

There is renewed scientific interest in the role of the immune system—especially that of T cell lymphocytes—in chronic fatigue syndrome. At this stage of knowledge, you should be evaluated at a university medical center and thereby avoid unnecessary and expensive diagnostic tests, as well as potentially harmful treatment procedures.

Theories have come and gone regarding the cause of this syndrome. Epstein-Barr virus (the cause of mononucleosis) was thought to be important. Candida and yeast infections were implicated. Group hysteria has explained some "outbreaks."

Chronic fatigue syndrome is most frequently diagnosed in young adult women. As many as 80% of patients with this diagnosis also are allergic and suffer from hay fever, asthma, and/or sinusitis. Many will, of course, benefit from allergy treatment. We stress that patients and physicians must first consider and rule out other illnesses for which fatigue is a frequent symptom. In addition to allergy, these include hypothyroidism, anemia, autoimmune disease, cancer, and chronic infections (Lyme disease, prostate tumor).

IF IT ISN'T ASTHMA, WHY AM I SHORT OF BREATH?

One morning we received a call from a nearby medical office. We had been treating the receptionist for hives. Her coworker explained that she had developed acute hives in the office and was wheezing so badly she couldn't talk. She was rushed to our office. The patient had obvious hives, loud and stridorous wheezing, and could only speak in short phrases. The wheezes occurred mainly on inspiration (breathing in), however, and no mucus sounds were heard in her chest. Her lips were pink, not blue. Offering reassurance only, this severe and frightening episode resolved and a saline aerosol mist relieved associated dry throat.

The diagnosis is vocal cord dysfunction—a condition often confused with asthma. In an attack the vocal cords come together as the patient inspires, obstructing the air flow. He or she can't speak and is hoarse. Sometimes direct visualization of the vocal cords during an attack is necessary to firmly confirm the diagnosis. The stress of our patient's new outbreak of hives had precipitated an attack of vocal cord dysfunction. This condition even can affect children, and sometimes teenage athletes suffer severe attacks under the stress of competition.

The treatment for vocal cord dysfunction is the use of relaxation, mindfulness exercises, and breathing techniques. Speech therapists can teach the patient to use abdominal breathing and allow the vocal cords to open. Failure to diagnose and treat vocal cord dysfunction can subject the patient to much unnecessary asthma medication, including prednisone.

WHAT IS CANDIDA?

Candida is a yeast normally found in the gastrointestinal tract and vaginas of healthy individuals. Overgrowth of this organism can cause disease in certain circumstances: AIDS; antibiotic use in women, vaginitis; inhaled steroids for asthma, throat involvement; and even diaper rashes. Ordinarily, however, we all live in harmony with this potentially dangerous yeast organism.

Some patients with "Candida" have reported a multiplicity of symptoms that have no discernible cause. These may include weakness, headache, anxiety, and difficulty with concentration, in addition to hay fever and bronchial asthma. Candida hypersensitivity has been inappropriately blamed. These complaints in fact are not related to each other in a recognized illness syndrome, and there is no evidence that they are caused by Candida. Candida treatment has not been shown to be helpful; and, in fact, some anti-Candida medications can be dangerous for allergic patients.

ARE MY HEADACHES FROM ALLERGY?

They may be. However, before investigating possible food or inhalant allergies, you should have your physician or a neurologist evaluate other possible serious causes of headache.

Sometimes the typical migraine headache responds to treatment with an elimination diet. Selected allergy testing for foods may guide your allergy specialist. These may be common or uncommon food allergens that are diagnosed by history, skin testing, and trial elimination diet regimens. If you are allergic to mold spores, you may want to try the mold-free diet. Certain foods result in high levels of the amino acid tyramine and these can trigger your migraines—chocolate, cheese, fermented foods, beer, wine, liver, yeast, yogurt, sausage, broad beans, and caffeine. Foods with high serotonin and salicylate levels have been suspect. Banana, red plum, tomato, avocado, potato, spinach, raspberry, eggplant, and nuts, especially walnuts, should also be considered.

Another type of headache that may clear after food elimination is the "histamine" or "cluster" headache, which is usually located on only one side of the head and is associated with tearing from the eye on the same side. The most common headache—the "tension headache" or myogenic headache—may also be caused by food allergies. In this case, a carefully followed regimen of food elimination and subsequent challenge testing will often provide the important diagnostic clues. The cause of a "sinus headache" is usually the same inhalant factor (pollen, dust, mold) or food that is causing the stuffy nose and sneezing that often accompany this type of headache. Sinus infection should always be considered.

CAN "FAD" DIETS AFFECT MY HEALTH?

Yes. Fad diets, such as unbalanced macrobiotic and fruitarian regimens, often eliminate important and necessary nutrients. Some dieters have experienced excessive weight loss and protein deficiency, leading to poor health. Food allergy sufferers need special guidance in order to avoid their allergenic foods while at the same time achieving appropriate nutrition. Bean and nut allergies present a special problem for sensitive vegetarian patients. Vitamin and mineral deficiencies may also occur. There have been recent reports of rickets in children who are fed only "natural" unfortified foods and, at the same time, do not get adequate sunlight for vitamin D.

SHOULD I FAST?

Prolonged fasting is dangerous and is not advised. Such extreme elimination of all foods is not necessary for the careful investigation of food allergy, which can be best accomplished by the strict trial elimination of selected foods for three weeks at a time. Subsequent challenges with the eliminated foods will then either absolve them or confirm their roles as the cause of symptoms.

A modified fast for a limited determined period entailing the use of a nonallergenic nutrient substitute such as Tolerex might be of benefit when ordinary methods for the diagnosis of suspected food allergy have failed. After all potential allergy-evoking foods are eliminated, the responsible allergen can then be clearly identified when it is re-introduced into the diet. This test, however, *must* be done only under the close supervision of your physician.

CAN DIET HELP MY HYPERACTIVE CHILD?

Behavioral changes have been observed to result from ingesting allergenic foods. These changes are known as the allergic tension–fatigue syndrome. Your child may become more irritable, anxious, or excessively tired. The appearance of facial pallor, dark circles around the eyes, and complaints about stomachaches and headaches are all part of this syndrome. Symptoms are improved during the course of a proper elimination diet designed to identify the offending foods.

Controlled studies have shown that food colorings at high doses—particularly FD&C No. 5 tartrazine yellow—exacerbate hyperactivity in 5% of "hyperactive" children. Hyperactive behavior is a manifestation of the larger syndrome called ADD (attention-deficit disorder) or ADHD (attention-deficit hyperactivity disorder). Though food additives do not cause this problem, there can be no harm in a trial elimination of unnecessary food coloring from the diet; however, it is a mistake to primarily ascribe any aspect of ADD to foods. There are no reports of adequate control of ADD by diet manipulation and while you are inappropriately focusing on the diet you may be wasting valuable time that should be spent on family counseling as well as psychological and medical management.

CAN SUGAR CAUSE ALLERGY?

Sugars do not cause allergy. Chemically, sugars are called *saccharides*. Glucose and fructose are found in fruits and vegetables; they are called simple sugar units or *monosaccharides*. Fructose is the very sweet sugar found in honey. Sucrose, the sugar found in cane and beets, is a compound of glucose and fructose and is termed a *disaccharide*. Lactose, the sugar of milk, is a combination of glucose and a unique milk sugar, galactose. Milk sugar and sucrose must be broken down to the simple monosaccharides before they can be absorbed from the intestines.

A current fad considers honey (fructose) to be natural and refined or purified sucrose from sugar cane as unnatural. Actually, both are equally natural. When you eat cane sugar, the body absorbs the digested products, glucose and fructose.

When many sugar units are joined together by plants or bacteria, starch and polysaccharides are formed. Only certain polysaccharides are commonly found in the cell walls of bacteria and can act as antigens, causing the body to form antibodies. Starch and other polysaccharides have not been shown to cause the formation of allergy antibodies; neither have the mono- or disaccharides. Thus, sugar and other polysaccharides play no role in allergy.

CAN VITAMINS HELP MY ALLERGY?

Taking large amounts of common vitamins will not prevent or help allergies; nevertheless, the surface linings of your mucous membranes (especially those in the throat and nose) benefit from adequate vitamin intake. There is a resurgence of studies regarding vitamin supplementation. The antioxidant vitamins C, E, A, and its precursor, beta-carotene are currently being studied to determine their roles in the prevention of cancer, aging, and heart disease.

WHAT IS BEE POLLEN?

Bee pollen is pollen extracted from the surface of bee extremities. It is high in protein content and is sold in health food stores. When we looked at bee pollen samples under the microscope, we saw some broken parts of bee bodies. Some bee pollens share similar components with the allergenic pollen that we breathe. Severe allergic attacks and even anaphylaxis have been reported in pollen-sensitive individuals after they ingest bee pollen.

CAN I BE ALLERGIC TO CHLORINATED WATER?

Chlorine is not an allergen. Therefore, it cannot induce new allergies. Chlorine can, however, provoke symptoms that mimic allergies. It can irritate your eyes, nasal mucosa, and the skin lesions of your eczema whenever you swim in improperly chlorinated water. It can even make you sneeze! Actually, if your eyes are red and burning, the water in the pool probably has an inadequate amount of protective free chlorine, which results in a buildup of irritating chlorosamines. Improper pH acid–base balance can also cause eye irritation. If your swimming pool has a strong "chlorine" odor, it is caused by the chlorosamines and, in fact, the water may not be properly sanitized.

WHAT ABOUT GINSENG?

An ancient Chinese monk once commented,

> "Ginseng will convey you with the speed of the wind to the grotto of eternal spring. It will give your loins twofold, nay, tenfold vigor, anchor your teeth more firmly, and increase the keenness of your sight."

This prized herb, which is extracted from a root of the plant panax, has been used by the Chinese for over 4000 years. It is used to revitalize, as well as to treat asthma and such disorders as diabetes and sexual impotence.

Scientists have studied the herb and found it to contain several pharmacologically active substances (panaxin, panax acid, and pancen) that increase body metabolism and stimulate a number of organs, including the heart and nervous system.

There are different types of ginseng: *Panax quinquefolia* (American) and *Panax ginseng* (Korean, Chinese). The Eastern type is rare and very expensive. The American type is more plentiful and less expensive, but it is less potent.

Beware of drug interactions and the side effects of herbal preparations. Some contain unknown amounts of ephedrine, which can dangerously raise blood pressure and cause agitation if you are susceptible, whereas others may contain a variety of potentially toxic ingredients. The State of California Department of Health Services has a list of "common toxic ingredients found in Asian patent medicines" (*see* box on opposite page).

Historically, many of our most useful drugs have herbal origins. In fact, the first effective medication for asthma utilized in Western countries was discovered in China, Ma Huang, which

---

**COMMON TOXIC INGREDIENTS FOUND
IN ASIAN PATENT MEDICINES**

- Cinnabar or calomel, contains a mercury compound
- Orpiment or realgar, contains arsenic
- Litharge and minium, contains lead oxide
- Borneol, a toxic chemical
- Aconite or aconitum, a toxic plant
- Bufonis venemum (toad secretion), secretions from certain toads
- Mylabris, a toxic insect
- Scorpion or buthus, toxic whole bodies of scorpions
- Borax, a toxic chemical
- Acorax, plant containing toxic chemicals
- Strychnos nux vomica or semen strychni, toxic seeds

Source: State of California Department of Health Services.

---

was later synthesized in Germany as ephedrine. Current studies are looking at scutellaria root, which is now known to inhibit the release of histamine and leukotrienes, and whose decoction is used to treat allergies.

WHAT ABOUT CAMOMILE TEA?

Drinking camomile tea is a popular folk cure for respiratory illness and flu in Western European cultures. Interestingly, camomile is in the ragweed family and serious allergic reactions to it have been reported. If you have a ragweed allergy, you should *not* drink camomile tea.

IS ARTHRITIS AN ALLERGY?

Many causes of the arthritis that produces joint changes have been discovered, and allergy is not among them. Arthritics suffering from severe allergies may feel general sickness or malaise and their joints may ache (arthralgia), but they do not develop any long-lasting disability or deformity. Fibromyalgia syndrome may be considered in those who do develop such joint problems.

WHAT IS FIBROMYALGIA SYNDROME?

Fibromyalgia syndrome is a condition of muscle soreness and tenderness, not arthritis. It is a form of rheumatism that does not affect your joints. Generalized pain is the most prominent complaint, and this pain may be quite severe in some. Your examination may give normal results, except for the finding of points of tenderness at your neck, shoulders, elbows, and knees. Your other complaints will often include fatigue and difficulty sleeping, depression, headaches, and abdominal discomfort. Your laboratory blood studies will be normal, so that the diagnosis is ultimately made from your history and physical examination. A variety of factors may cause this syndrome. It is not an allergy specifically, but there is an association with severe hay fever. When your hay fever is severe, you may feel excessive fatigue and your sleep will often be disturbed; you awaken with blocked nasal passages and a dry mouth. This sleep disturbance may explain the association between fibromyalgia and allergy. Your specific allergies should of course be treated, but most fibromyalgia patients are not allergic, and the mechanism or course of the syndrome is thought to be disruption of deep, restful sleep (REM). Your REM sleep may be restored by such medications as amitriptyline (Elavil) and doxepin (Sinequan), and additional important therapies including exercise, diet, meditation, and education.

WHAT IS PETROCHEMICAL ALLERGY?

Petrochemicals are the various hydrocarbons distilled from petroleum. They are potentially potent toxins; that is, in various concentrations, they can cause illness in all people. The fumes of these chemicals, such as gasoline, can give you headaches, malaise, and nausea, and in high concentrations they can be fatal. Altered immune reactions (allergy) to these substances have not, however, been reported.

Why Do Hair Sprays, Insect Sprays, and Air Fresheners Make My Allergy Worse?

Hair sprays contain chemical irritants that trigger the allergic response, but neither hair sprays nor the chemicals in air fresheners and cleaning preparations cause allergies as such. However, they can cause your allergic symptoms of nasal congestion or wheezing to flare up. You are more susceptible to these irritants precisely because you are allergic; your allergic mucous membranes are far more prone to react than those of a nonallergic individual.

Should I Get a Room Ionizer?

The ionizer generates charged particles called *negative ions* into the air; these negative ions bind onto particulate matter, thus forming larger and heavier particles that then settle to the ground.

This sounds like a good idea, but room ionizers have not been proven especially beneficial in treating allergies. They may remove allergenic particles such as dust and pollens from a small area surrounding the machine itself, but they do not provide sufficiently wide environmental control.

Will Meditation Help My Allergy?

It may help. Meditation resolves psychic and physical stress, factors that definitely aggravate your allergic status. This therapy has been practiced for hundreds of years by scholars and mystics in Europe and India. Current research on neurotransmitters is uncovering the chemicals in the brain and nervous system that directly affect our bodies and immune systems.

Airway resistance in asthma and vascular dilatation in allergic rhinitis are partially under the control of the autonomic (involuntary) nervous system. Meditation may modify this autonomic balance and thus give some symptomatic relief.

Mastering a meditation technique can be very helpful. When you first begin to wheeze, avoid panic and take your medicine immediately. Then sit down in a quiet area, close your eyes, and let your mind take you to a safe place which you have previously identified. This mental sanctuary might be the library of your high school or the home of your best friend. Then have your mind bring a spiritual advisor into that place, usually an old teacher, friend, or parent. Let your new spiritual advisor converse with you in an effort to get in touch with your real feelings. This entire process should be limited to 15–20 minutes maximum, after which you should be experiencing a sense of well-being with increased energy and tranquility, as well as easier breathing.

Do I Have to Sit Still to Meditate?

No. You can easily meditate and still mindfully engage in such ordinary activity as walking. The key is to focus intentionally on the elemental aspects of the activity—the movement of your legs on the ground, your breathing. This will allow you to achieve a different level of consciousness, and thereby get in touch with your inner self. You may actually be able to watch your thought processes arise, develop, and subside without "acting out" the old, tired patterns of behavior that flare asthma and allergy as well as ulcers and headaches.

Should I Seek Acupuncture Treatment?

Some allergy patients may feel relief with acupuncture and this has been successfully used as an adjunct therapy in selected cases, where the improvement of nasal and sinus symptoms is reported. The therapeutic effects ascribed to acupuncture treatment, however, may in fact be caused by your concurrent medications, such as a cortisone shot, and not by the acupuncture itself.

What Are Urine Shots?

Believe it or not, some attempt has been made to treat allergies by injecting patients with their own urine. We can't imagine the rationale for this useless and potentially dangerous procedure. Moreover, it is known that experimental rabbits injected with their own urine will develop severe kidney disease. *Don't be a guinea pig!*

10

Where Do I Go from Here?

Can I Diagnose Allergies Myself?
Which Allergies Can I Treat by Myself?
How Can I Control My Environment?
Must I Really Remove the Carpet?
Are There Special Vacuum Cleaners for Allergy?
Can Mites Be Exterminated?
Are Natural Foods Important?
Will an Air Filter Help?
Should I Take a Vacation During Pollen Season?
How Can I Build Up My Wind?
Will Breathing Exercises Help My Asthma?
At What Point Should I See an Allergist?
How Do I Choose an Allergist?
Will Insurance Provide for My Allergy Care?
How Much Will Allergy Consultation Cost?
What Are Some Sources for Ongoing Information
    Regarding Allergy and Asthma Care?

CAN I DIAGNOSE ALLERGIES MYSELF?

A keen observer often can! You can start by focusing on conditions and situations that may aggravate your allergy symptoms. For example, if your symptoms are worse indoors, at night, and there are early morning sneezing attacks, then you should suspect house dust or mold allergy, especially in moist and sheltered environments. Do you notice that symptoms are worse when you come home to your dog or cat, and improve when you leave? Are you symptom-free outdoors? Did you check your pillows for feathers?

If your hay fever is always worse on the golf course, then grass pollen is the most likely offender. If you get hives from peanuts, your allergy is obvious and strict avoidance is necessary. You know to avoid nickel in jewelry if you develop a rash on your pierced ears.

WHICH ALLERGIES CAN I TREAT BY MYSELF?

The best treatment of allergy always includes self-help. Avoidance is consistently the preferred form of therapy. If you are sensitive, don't visit parks and roll on the grass during April, May, and June—and postpone that camping trip until after the pollen season. If your sneezing, watery eyes, and wheezing are worse around dogs and cats, put them outside and don't visit homes with indoor pets. If cats cannot be removed from your home, you can significantly reduce the amount of cat allergen by washing your cat every one to two weeks. Regular vacuuming is essential for the removal of cat allergen, but steam cleaning provides no additional help. Even after the cat has been removed, it takes six months before the level of cat allergen is reduced to a level comparable to that found in homes that have never had a cat. Effective house dust mite and mold control measures can be carried out by sensitive patients and these procedures are extremely important for successful overall management of your allergies.

Adequate rest—sometimes just an extra hour of sleep—and good nutrition are most important. These simple measures are often very helpful.

Take an antihistamine like Chlor-Trimeton if you are in an unavoidable allergic circumstance. It may be all that is necessary to ward off disturbing and uncomfortable symptoms. Be aware of the many medications available over-the-counter.

If you develop asthma—a more serious problem—follow your asthma control plan with appropriate prescribed medications. Intal or nedocromil, and/or inhaled steroids and, if necessary, albuterol will give you significant relief. Of course, if you have an unforeseen attack and you are without your prescribed medication, Primatene mist or Bronkaid inhalers will usually give you fast but very temporary relief.

How Can I Control My Environment?

For House Dust Mites

The bedroom should be given first priority because you spend approximately six to ten hours a day breathing the air in that room. When you lie down in bed or on the couch or carpet, you breathe in as much as 100 times more mite allergen as you would when standing. Mites feed on human dander—the proteinaceous flecks of skin you are constantly shedding. The dust mites are not parasites—they are never on your body. They live on the surfaces of your mattress, blankets, pillows, comforters, and your sofa. The carpet is an important reservoir for breeding mites and danders.

House dust mite control measures include the following:

- Cover *all mattresses and box springs* in your bedroom with zippered vinyl encasings. Strong and very comfortable vinyl laminated encasings can be obtained from Allergy Control Products, Inc., 96 Danbury Road, Ridgefield, Connecticut 06877.
- A mattress pad is necessary and makes the mattress encasings comfortable; this mattress pad should be washed in the hot water cycle of the washing machine every two weeks.
- Vacuum the mattresses and areas around and underneath the beds, including the closets, once a week; not more often. Wiping off the mattress with a damp cloth and daily wet mopping of the floors is very effective.

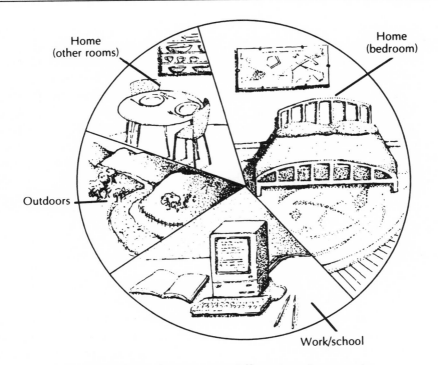

Portion of the day spent in different environments.

- All bedding including bedspreads, comforters, and pillows should be washed periodically. Again, the hot water cycle (temperature of greater than 130 degrees) is essential for killing the dust mites and denaturing the protein allergen for sheets and pillow cases as well as all other bedding.
- Bare vinyl or hardwood floors, and windows without draperies are best, although small washable rugs and curtains may be used.
- Remove upholstered furniture, stuffed toys, books and bookcases, and other dust-collecting items from the bedroom. Dacron or foam rubber may be substituted for the potential dust-producing material that is commonly found in stuffed toys. It takes only a moment of sewing.
- House dust mite-allergic individuals should also avoid down and feathers—check your pillows, comforters, and clothing.

> ### MOLD "HOT SPOTS"
>
> - Bathroom and kitchen sink areas; behind refrigerators, around showers, tubs, toilets; cabinets and floor areas
> - Mattresses and box springs, especially the underside surfaces; and foam rubber mattresses
> - Walls, especially old wallpaper and wallpaper behind furniture, desks, bookcases (use mold-inhibiting paints)
> - Under porches and basement areas
> - Closets
> - Garden and yard areas (piles of leaves)
> - Indoor household plants (remove them from the bedroom and place fine gravel over the soil)
> - Washing machine area—vent the dryer outdoors
> - Wicker baskets, carpet padding, humidifiers, air conditioners

- Placing a filter in the heater vent in your bedroom may be helpful. An air filter with a special HEPA filter can remove airborne dust, mold spores, and pollens. Central heating filters should be cleaned or replaced. If you use a humidifier in the winter, avoid excessive humidification and monitor the humidity. Try to keep the level at less than 50% humidity.

FOR MOLDS

An ordinary chlorine bleach, such as Clorox, is effective for eradicating molds and mildew. Lysol is also a good household cleansing agent. A dehumidifier may keep the humidity under 35% and thereby inhibit mold production.

Recognize "hot spots" where molds are most likely to accumulate (*see* box). Damp and sheltered environments encourage mold growth.

MUST I REALLY REMOVE THE CARPET?

Yes. If you have asthma or severe nasal and sinus symptoms and your dust mite allergy is a principal cause. This is not so difficult if there are wood floors under the carpeting. If you have to install a wood or vinyl floor, this can be costly. But remember, the most important place in your house is the bedroom because you spend 6–8 hours a day there. Additionally, children often play on the carpeted floor.

You must tailor your environmental control to the severity of your allergy problem. If your symptoms are mild to moderate, first try the other fundamental dust control measures. Make your efforts reasonable and not complicated and guilt-provoking.

ARE THERE SPECIAL VACUUM CLEANERS FOR ALLERGY?

You should use a tank vacuum with an exhaust filter or use a high efficiency vacuum bag. Do not vacuum more than once a week or you will stir up the dust mite particles too often. If the patient has to vacuum, a dust mask can be helpful, as will leaving the house for a few hours when the cleaning is done. Remember, mites thrive in high humidity and we do not recommend water-containing vacuums. It is reported that the exhaust vapors from the water actually contain dust mite extract.

CAN MITES BE EXTERMINATED?

A recent study reported that almost all houses of dust mite asthmatics across the country had mite antigen levels high enough to cause asthma. If your young child is allergic to mites, you can be sure that the exposure is coming from your home.

Mites cannot be permanently exterminated. Mite eggs are found wherever there are people and adherent surfaces such as carpets, clothing, bedding, and sofas. An acaracide—Acarosan (benzyl benzoate)—will kill the mites and can be applied to surfaces. It is not available as yet in California. There is also a solution with tannic acid (the same chemical found in small amounts in tea) that inactivates the mite allergenic particles. It is called Allergy Control Solution and can be sprayed directly on surfaces and it may stain. The solution should be used about every three months.

ARE NATURAL FOODS IMPORTANT?

Yes, but only for a small percentage of allergy patients. Some individuals experience allergic symptoms after eating foods containing colorings, preservatives, and other additives. Foods you prepare yourself will not contain these possible offenders. A strict trial elimination diet that uses only natural foods may be helpful.

If your symptoms subside with a natural food diet, you will be able to buy good products in most supermarkets. But remember, foods labeled "natural" or "organic" may still contain a variety of additives. Take the time to read labels carefully.

WILL AN AIR FILTER HELP?

Breathing cleaner air has given many hay fever and asthma sufferers good relief. This can be achieved by installing air-cleaning machines with special filters.

Choosing the right air cleaner or filter is important. High efficiency particulate air (HEPA) filters have been demonstrated to be effective in trapping most airborne allergens, such as pollen, mold, and house dust particles. The filter material is made of tiny glass fibers interfolded to allow the entrapment of small particles as the air is filtered through it. This filter is an important component in several commercial air cleaners. Prices for an air cleaner vary according to the size and model. The air cleaner can be adjusted to any room, although the bedroom should deserve first priority. An average bedroom air cleaner lists for around $300, but is frequently discounted. One patient with severe mold asthma, who lives in a damp environment in San Francisco, finally purchased a HEPA filter for his bedroom for under $200 and it has changed his life. He now uses much less medication, and is more comfortable in his daily life.

Another type of air cleaner utilizes an electrostatic precipitator device that magnetically traps charged particles. A major disadvantage of such a system is that some models emit ozone. Ozone levels at 0.3 ppm (parts per million by volume of air) can

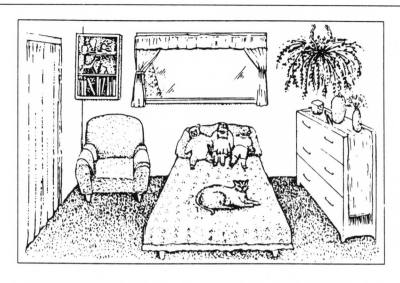

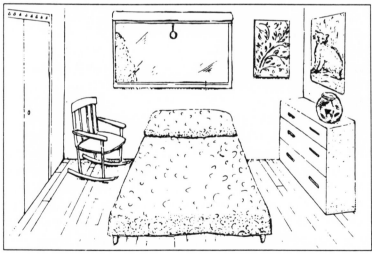

Allergenic room (top) and nonallergenic room (bottom).

precipitate coughing and choking, thus making your asthma worse. Lower levels cause nasal and eye irritation.

An air cleaner may be rented first to evaluate its effectiveness. Stores will often credit the customer's rental costs toward the purchase cost.

SHOULD I TAKE A VACATION DURING POLLEN SEASON?

Yes. You may have trouble deducting it as a medical expense, but a vacation during a short two- to three-week pollen season could be a very effective treatment for your allergies. The difficulty with this includes the time you may have to be away and the distance that may be necessary to travel. You may also just trade your ragweed symptoms for other severe pollen or mold allergies in the vacation area.

Immunotherapy with allergy shots will provide relief 90% of the time. This is far more reliable and realistic than island hopping all year.

HOW CAN I BUILD UP MY WIND?

You can "build up your wind" with an exercise program that becomes progressively more strenuous. This is actually aerobic exercise, which utilizes oxygen and makes you become a more efficient breather. If such a program is followed regularly, your breathing will become less labored with activities and exertion. A person who is aerobically fit can much better tolerate an exacerbation of asthma.

We encourage asthmatic patients to participate in sports activities, especially swimming. Other aerobic exercises, such as jogging, bicycling, long walks, ballet, jazz exercise, stepping exercises, and stationary bicycling are excellent. Indoor exercise has advantages for asthmatics, especially during smog alerts and the pollen season. Additionally, if wheezing flares you can relax and be in a safe place. You can also benefit from "pumping iron" and other regulated weight programs such as the Nautilus type of circuit-weight training. Upper arm and shoulder muscle development is important.

WILL BREATHING EXERCISES HELP MY ASTHMA?

Breathing exercises teach efficient breathing and relaxation; you will learn the technique of diaphragmatic breathing— using the diaphragm to take in more air.

These techniques are not necessary for most asthmatics, but may be helpful for panic-stricken children who suffer frequent attacks. Breathing exercises should not and cannot be a substitute for a complete asthma control plan.

AT WHAT POINT SHOULD I SEE AN ALLERGIST?

When your symptoms are inadequately controlled in spite of all your efforts at self-help, you should seek medical advice. Your primary care physician can often help you evaluate and manage the problem. Consultation with an allergy/asthma specialist may be necessary to detect allergens that may have escaped your notice and to plan the best treatment. If your symptoms are severe and you need allergy immunotherapy injections, the special training and experience of an allergist is necessary. Only patients with significant allergies require shots, and of course the most appropriate use of the new, potent allergy extracts for treatment requires the expertise of a specialist. Additionally, an allergist is especially helpful with the often difficult task of developing a comprehensive asthma control plan.

HOW DO I CHOOSE AN ALLERGIST?

The best way to choose an allergist is to ask your primary care physician or the local medical society for a referral to a physician certified by the American Board of Allergy and Immunology. Then make inquiries about your candidate allergist(s) among other physicians as well as community professionals and friends. Alternatively, you might ask the candidates' office receptionist by phone not only about the physician's board certification and training in allergy, but also about his or her medical school faculty appointments, and activity in local allergy societies. Remember that membership or fellowship in a professional specialty society is not the same as board certification in that specialty. Satisfactory replies to all the above do not always guarantee success in your choice of an allergist; nevertheless, they are most helpful guidelines.

Certification by the American Board of Allergy and Immunology currently requires completion of a two-year postgraduate fellowship in allergy and immunology, as well as complete specialty training and board certification in either pediatrics or internal medicine. After training, a new physician must pass a difficult qualifying examination that encompasses all phases of allergy and immunology, including asthma and other chest diseases, aerobiology, and skin disorders.

Finally, interpersonal relationships, though intangible, are always important in the doctor–patient relationship. If you feel you cannot communicate comfortably with your allergist, a change is necessary.

WILL INSURANCE PROVIDE FOR MY ALLERGY CARE?

Your coverage will vary greatly depending on the contract with your medical health plan. If you are considering an HMO, PPO, or other managed care plan, make sure you select one that allows you access to a board-certified allergy specialist as well as other necessary specialty care.

HOW MUCH WILL ALLERGY CONSULTATION COST?

Your out-of-pocket cost will depend on your insurance. There are often copayments and deductibles. Most allergists work under contract with insurance companies, and reimbursements are fixed for consultations, office visits, and procedures. Especially if you are not insured or have high deductibles, make sure that you, as the patient, together with your doctor, establish the goals of the consultation and the costs for each component. Consultation that includes taking a detailed history and physical is most important and valuable. Additional costs reflect the need for allergy skin testing. In California with its pollen seasons during most months of the year, allergy evaluation requires approximately 100 prick-scratch tests and perhaps 25 intradermal tests. If food tests are indicated, the number should be based on your history. Remember, the majority of food allergies are caused by fewer than 20 foods. Special circumstances exist with drug allergy and insect sting allergy, where costs are increased based on observation time and the expense of the allergy test materials. Additionally, spirometry is necessary for the evaluation and continuing management of all patients with asthma symptoms. Fees vary greatly with geographic location.

It is impossible to compare the value of personal professional services. Variables include the availability of the allergist, the allergist's qualifications, the time spent with you the patient, and the complexity of your specific allergy.

WHAT ARE SOME SOURCES FOR ONGOING INFORMATION REGARDING ALLERGY AND ASTHMA CARE?

National Asthma Network
Mothers of Asthmatics
Suite 200
3554 Chainbridge Road
Fairfax, VA 22030
Phone: 800-878-4403

American Academy of Allergy and Immunology
611 East Wells Street
Milwaukee, WI 53202
Phone: 414-272-6071 or 800-822-2762

American College of Allergy and Immunology
85 West Algonquin, Suite 550
Arlington Heights, IL 60005
Phone: 312-359-2800 or 800-842-7777

National Jewish Center for Immunology
   and Respiratory Medicine
1400 Jackson Street
Denver, CO 80206
Phone: 303-398-1079 or 800-222-5864

Local Chapters of the American Lung Association
   or American Lung Association
1740 Broadway
New York, NY 11229
Phone: 212-315-8700

Asthma and Allergy Foundation of America
1125 15th Street, N.W., Suite 502
Washington, DC 20005
Phone: 800-727-8462

National Asthma Education Program
4733 Bethesda Avenue
Bethesda, MD 20815
Phone: 301-251-1222

National Heart, Lung and Blood Institute
NIH Building 31, Room 4A21
9000 Rockville Pike
Bethesda, MD 20892
Phone: 301-496-4236

Glossary

AIDS: An illness caused by the Human Immunodeficiency Virus (HIV) that destroys the CD4⁺ T-cells and damages the immune defense system.

Adrenalin (epinephrine): A powerful hormone that relaxes bronchial muscles, stimulates the heart, and is necessary for the treatment of severe allergic reactions.

Allergen: Substance (usually a protein) that causes the formation of allergy antibodies and/or sensitized cells in your body, and subsequently triggers the allergic response.

Allergy shots: Specific immunotherapy used for pollens, dust mites, animal danders, and molds.

Anaphylaxis: A severe and immediate allergic reaction—it may include hives, trouble breathing, loss of blood pressure (shock), or all three.

Angioedema: Swelling of various body parts, especially around the eyes and lips.

Antibody: A serum protein that fights infection or causes allergy.

Antihistamine: The most commonly used drug for allergies; blocks histamines and thereby lessens allergic response.

Anti-inflammatory agents: With reference to asthma, drugs that diminish swelling, edema, and cellular infiltration. They are usually necessary for treatment and reduce the need for bronchodilators.

Arterial gas embolism: A large bubble of air carried from the lungs to the brain.

Asthma: Inflammation and spasm of the bronchial tubes.

211

Asthma control plan: The patient and physician agree to specific actions to improve the quality of life by first avoiding the causes of, and then treating, asthma.

Bronchitis: Inflammation or infection of the bronchial tubes in the lungs.

Bronchodilator: Medication that relaxes the spasm of the bronchial tubes in asthma.

Bronchospasm: Constriction of the airways (bronchial tubes).

Celiac disease: Diarrhea and malabsorption of food caused by intolerance to gluten, a protein of wheat, rye, oats, and barley.

Cholinergic urticaria: Tiny hives caused by heat and exercise.

Conjunctivae: The inner linings of the eyelid and the covering of the eyeball.

Cortisone: An important steroid used to treat severe allergic reactions.

Dander: Flecks of skin that are shed by pets and people; a frequent cause of allergy and food for mites.

Decongestant: The ingredient in an allergy medication that constricts blood vessels and reduces the swelling that causes congestion.

Eczema: An itchy and dry skin rash, often caused by allergy.

Emphysema: A destructive disease of the lungs, which sometimes has a reversible asthmatic component.

Eosinophils: Special white blood cells important in allergic inflammation.

Gammaglobulins: Antibodies belonging to various classes—IgG, IgM, IgA, and IgE—which variously fight infections and also cause immune disorders such as allergy.

Histamine: A chemical substance, released by mast cells, that causes the allergic symptoms of itching, swelling, and bronchial spasms.

Immune system: The machinery in your body that recognizes and reacts to foreign materials such as pollens, cat dander, bacteria, and viruses.

Immunotherapy: Treatment with injections of allergy-causing substances in order to desensitize allergy patients to the specific inhalants and/or medication to which they are sensitive.

Inflammation: The body's response process to foreign substances or injury in which multiple cells gather and release chemical mediators, resulting in swelling and damage of body tissue.

Intradermal testing: Allergy skin tests performed by the injection of allergens into the skin.

Leukotrienes: Cellular chemical mediators of the allergic response, especially asthma.

Lymphocytes: White blood cells that produce antibodies and regulate the immune response.

Mast cells: Cells containing histamine and other mediators such as leukotrienes; found in the mucous membranes, bronchial tubes, and skin. Basophils in the blood have some common characteristics and similarly participate in the allergic reaction.

Mindfulness exercises: Disciplines of self-awareness and "going inward" to deal with stress and disease—yoga, tai-chi, meditation.

Mold: A minute fungus—for instance, mildew—that causes allergy by producing airborne spores.

Mucous membranes: The moist linings of the mouth, nose, and other parts of the respiratory, digestive, and reproductive systems.

Nasal polyp: Fluid-laden outpouchings from the lining of the sinuses; not tumors.

Oral allergy syndrome: Itchiness of the mouth from certain allergenic foods such as kiwi, peaches, and melons.

Peak flow meter: A small and handy device to monitor your asthma by measuring your expiratory flow rate.

Pollens: Tiny plant grains (15–60 microns) carrying the male reproductive parts that fertilize the female plant ovary and thereby produce a seed.

Skin testing: A diagnostic technique in which a small amount of antigen is introducedinto the skin by prick/puncture or injection. A local reaction is measured.

Spores: The very tiny (1 micron) reproductive parts of a mold (fungus).

Steroids: Hormones, such as cortisone, that regulate body functions and are produced by the endocrine glands. They are also pharmacological agents.

TMJ: Temporomandibular joint syndrome or dysfunction is a painful inflammation of the jaw joint.

Tracheostomy: A surgical procedure in which a cut is made through the neck to allow airflow to and from the lungs.

Urticaria: Hives or welts.

Venom: The poison of stinging insects, which contains allergens.

Index